SOMATIC THERAPY FOR THE MIND-BODY CONNECTION

A Beginner's Guide to Healing Trauma and Relieving Chronic Stress and Tension with Easy On-the-Go Psychosomatic Exercises

JESSICA STARLING

Table of Contents

particular purpose. No warranty may be created or extended by sales representatives or written sales materials. The advice and strategies contained herein may not be suitable for your situation. You should consult with a professional when appropriate.

The resources in this book are provided for informational purposes only and should not be used to replace the specialized training and professional judgment of a health care or mental health care professional.

Neither the publisher nor the author shall be liable for any loss of profit or any other commercial damages, including but not limited to special, incidental, consequential, personal, or other damages.

Somatic Therapy for the Mind-Body Connection
A Beginner's Guide to Healing Trauma and Relieving Chronic Stress and Tension with Easy On-the-Go Psychosomatic Exercises

By Jessica Starling

[ISBN] *only needed for print books*

ACKNOWLEDGMENTS

To many, this might be just a book, but to me, this is one of the biggest achievements of my life in my quest to improve my health alongside helping as many people as possible; so where do I start? I owe so much to so many. I wrote a list of people I'd like to mention as my way of saying thank you, and that list is huge. 10 people and 2 dogs long, so here goes. To my publishing mentors Chris and Angelina who guided me every step of the way, I thank you. I thank Ava Priestley, author of a book titled 'Small Talk. Big Impact', for putting up with my incessant messaging and always showing me kindness. Morag, for her commitment to helping me build my team of early readers who helped read, refine and improve this book in preparation for release on Amazon.

Trish and Ruth, both amazing Yoga teachers, whom I leaned on more than once for advice. All the brilliant hand-drawn illustrations by the amazing Susan Cotgreave (Instagram: @susan.elsie.studios).

The support I received from my life coach and now friend Gina. My brilliant friend Amy for her unwavering commitment to just being there. The unbelievable support from a very close friend Emily. I feel I would have failed without you. Last but not least, my two small dogs Nala and Kaiser. They have shared many tears with me. Thank you. And finally, also to you the reader, I thank you for purchasing this book and becoming one of my friends on this journey together. I hope from the bottom of my heart that you find the information I have included useful and helpful for whatever you may or may not be going through right now. I wish you all the strength to heal your mind, body and spirit.

AUTHORS FOREWORD

One childhood memory I have is sitting in the back of my mum and dad's car on a sunny day, passing a place where my mum used to work with horses, and her saying out loud that her old boss or friend (I can't remember) stopped talking to her and she had no idea why. I was about 8. Little did I know that this would be a theme throughout my life. Not only that, but when I was at my last job, I was the subject of psychological bullying. This made me very ill, and I acted like I didn't care, but I did as I never knew why it was happening. This is why I've chosen to write this book under a pen name, rather than use my own. For fear of certain people finding out who it is and subjecting me to further bullying for publishing a book on a topic I'm passionate about. This fear in me clearly still runs deep. At the back of this book, I mention Jessica is trying to help a friend who suffers from multiple sclerosis. Well, that person is her.

One day I'd like to tell you about the woman in the cafe and the light. A fascinating story that made my treatment at the hands of these people clear. But that is for another book.

INTRODUCTION

As we go through life, the stress of daily living can take its toll on us, particularly our own body. Most of the time, we don't even know it is happening. This undoubtedly will cause unnecessary stress, tension, and trauma. Within us all, lies the ability to bridge the gap between your mind and body making your life a whole lot easier. Let's face it, this is what we all want. Life is tough enough as it is, without your own body turning on you. This is what somatic therapy can achieve, taking you back to yourself.

"Somatic Therapy for the Mind-Body Connection" is more than just a book; it's a journey that doesn't require you to step away from your life. Nobody has time to stop and do anything these days, and you probably don't even know how important somatics is. This is why I've thought about on-the-go techniques. Whether you're new to somatics, or a seasoned pro, this book is designed to help you to keep moving forward with healing.

14

Together, we'll look at simple, yet powerful, on-the-go psychosomatic exercises and how they can be your best friend against the daily silent fight against trauma, stress, and tension. Through these pages, you will learn to survive, building resilience, emotional freedom, and a deeper, more joyful connection with your mind and body.

It will be a journey of discovery and healing, revealing what strength you really have that lies within you, and how it's accessible at any given moment, one breath, one movement, one heartbeat at a time. In today's world, we are constantly looking for new ways to heal and connect. Somatics isn't new, but it's often described with scientific jargon that none of us understand. So, let's try to understand it once and for all. Let us begin.

What this book does

Methods and Ideas that Work - In the book, you'll learn unique somatic exercises designed specifically for people with busy lifestyles, so you'll get new perspectives on well-known techniques.

On-the-go exercises - Almost every chapter has easy, accessible exercises. For individuals with busy schedules, these exercises can be seamlessly incorporated into daily routines, making somatics more accessible.

Getting in touch with your senses and self-aware-ness - This book emphasizes developing a rich sensory vocabulary and self-awareness. Readers will learn how to express emotions and sensations more clearly, which opens the body's inherent wisdom and healing power.

The use of narrative - To make the book engaging and relatable, many chapters begin with a narrative. They give you insight into the real-world potential impact that somatic practices can have on individuals.

Element of interaction - Self-inquiry exercises and reflection prompts encourage active participation. Using interactive elements, readers can take the concepts and apply them to their own lives.

Holistic Approach - Taking a holistic approach, the book addresses the emotional, physical, and spiritual aspects of healing and well-being. Readers are encouraged to explore the ways somatic practices can improve their health, relationships, and creativity.

Community and Connection - In the book, the author emphasizes the importance of community and social support. Providing guidance on how to find and form somatic practice groups, share experiences with others, and build supportive networks that enhance personal growth.

Commitment to Accessibility - The book is all about making somatic practices accessible, including to people with disabilities or new to bodywork. All exercises have been modified and adapted to make them inclusive and accessible.

With these elements incorporated, the book offers a comprehensive, engaging, and accessible guide to somatic therapy that can be used to explore the mind-body connection and heal.

Who can benefit from this book?

Through somatic exercises, EFT tapping, and Qigong integration, this book can help a wide range of people, including anyone experiencing stress and anxiety - With this book, you'll find practical tools and strategies for managing daily stress, reducing anxiety, and improving your mental health.

Individuals healing from trauma - There are several gentle, body-centered approaches outlined in this book that you can use to heal from past traumas, including tapping and somatic exercises.

Busy professionals - Featuring on-the-go exercises and mindfulness practices to fit into a busy schedule, this book is perfect for stress relief and balance for busy professionals.

Athletes and physical practitioners - By developing a deeper connection with their bodies, people can enhance body awareness, improve performance, and reduce the risk of injury.

People with chronic pain or illness-Long-term health conditions and chronic pain can be managed with these strategies.

Mindfulness practitioners and meditators - By practicing somatics and Qigong exercises, people can deepen their mindfulness practice and become more aware of their bodies.

Mental health professionals - It's a great resource for therapists, counsellors, and other mental health professionals who want to offer body-centered practices to help their clients heal.

Spiritual seekers - Those seeking inner peace, balance, and enlightenment might find the combination of body and mind practices useful.

Fitness and wellness enthusiasts - Its approach to combining physical health with emotional and spiritual well-being is perfect for anyone interested in holistic health, fitness, or wellness.

Generally, this book is suitable for anyone looking to enhance the quality of their life through accessi-

ble and practical techniques that bridge the gap between physical health and emotional wellness, promoting a deeper sense of connection between body
and mind.

How to use this book

For best results, read it from beginning to end to get
the whole picture. After you read it, think about how
these practices might benefit you, such as stress relief, trauma healing, or mindfulness. Rather than
overloading yourself with too many changes at
once, start small, adding just one or two exercises
into your daily routine. Keeping a journal can help
you keep track of your experiences, emotions, and
insights. This can help you track your progress and
get to know yourself better. If you have any physical
limitations or special needs, feel free to adapt the
exercises. The book isn't intended to be a strict
guide. Once you're comfortable with the initial techniques that you've chosen, gradually introduce new
practices from other chapters. Be sure to review the
material regularly to make sure you're still learning.

Talking about your journey with others can also be beneficial, giving you extra motivation. Above all, remember to be patient and kind to yourself. It takes time for healing and growth, and every small step forward is worth celebrating. Using this book and its practices with openness and self-compassion is the key to a better life

CHAPTER 1

Part 1

THE FOUNDATIONS OF SOMATIC THERAPY

Imagine stepping into a time machine, not to explore the outer reaches of our world, but to explore the mind-body connection. We would find out that somatics has always been around. From the meditative disciplines of the East to the holistic healing traditions of Indigenous cultures, the principles of somatics have been quietly shaping our understanding of health and wellness. Yet, somatics is not a past tradition; it is a living, breathing discipline that evolves with our growing understanding of human biology, psychology, and neurology.

Understanding somatics

The field of somatics focuses on how we perceive and experience our bodies. "Somatics" is a term coined by Thomas Hanna in the 1970s, coming from the Greek word "soma," which means the living body. Somatic practices are based on the idea

22

that your mind and body are one thing, with each improving the other.

Somatic practices are all about enhancing body awareness - awareness of your own body's state. The heightened awareness can help you release tension, correct poor posture, and move more efficiently. There are lots of practices under the somatics umbrella, including the Alexander Technique, Feldenkrais Method, Hakomi Method, and Body-Mind centering. They all have their own techniques and underlying philosophy, but they all work towards improving mind-body integration.

Benefits of somatic practices may include:

improved Posture and Movement - You can reduce strain and improve alignment and efficiency by becoming more aware of habits and patterns of movement and posture.

Reduction of pain-A lot of somatic practices are effective in managing and reducing chronic pain, especially muscular tension.

Stress Reduction - Mindfulness and bodily aware-ness can reduce stress levels and improve your mood.

A better mind-body connection - It's possible to deepen the relationship between physical sensations and emotional states with somatics, getting better psychological insight and balancing our emotions.

Improved flexibility and mobility - You can improve your flexibility and range of motion by moving gently and mindfully.

Better Balance and Coordination - Somatic practices can improve balance and coordination by refining body awareness.

Often people use somatics for rehabilitation, to improve their performance, or just to feel better. This is particularly beneficial for those who wish to develop a deeper understanding of the signals sent by their bodies to make informed decisions about how to respond to them.

At its heart lie these key principles:

The Mind-Body Connection: Somatics teaches us that the mind and body are not separate. They are a dynamic, interconnected system. Our thoughts, emotions, and beliefs can manifest physically, just as our bodily states can influence our mental and emotional well-being.

Self-awareness: Central to somatics is mindful awareness of the body's sensations, movements, and responses. This awareness is the first step toward healing and change.

Movement's Healing Power: Movement is both a language and a medicine. Somatic practices use gentle, intentional movements to release tension, process trauma, and restore balance to the mind-body system.

Being your own boss: Somatics lets individuals become active participants in their healing journey, offering tools for self-regulation, resilience, and autonomy.

25

Integration: The goal of somatics is not only to alleviate symptoms but to integrate our mind-body connection and bring physical, mental and emotional harmony.

As we explore somatics, remember that this journey is not about acquiring new techniques, but remembering and reclaiming what our bodies have known all along. So, let's take this journey with curiosity, openness, and readiness to explore the landscape of our inner worlds.

Part 2

This healing process can take the form of mindful relaxation, meditation, and other techniques that allow the body to restore its natural balance. It is important to remember that our bodies are designed to be resilient, and with the right tools and support, we can help them to heal and restore balance.

HOW TRAUMA AFFECTS THE BODY

In response to trauma, the body goes through a series of complex reactions. In the beginning, it triggers the fight-or-flight response, causing adrenaline and cortisol to be released. It's also possible for trauma to have long-term effects on the autonomic nervous system, which can throw off the balance between sympathetic and parasympathetic divisions, keeping you on edge all the time.

There is no doubt that these physiological changes are reflected by alterations in the brain itself, particularly the areas that are responsible for processing emotional information. Memory problems, and difficulties concentrating, can result from such changes. Physical health can deteriorate because of prolonged stress, including heart disease, digestion problems, and weakened immunity.

Trauma affects both your mind and body. Conditions like depression, anxiety, PTSD, substance abuse, and sleep disturbances can be caused by it. Trauma requires a holistic approach that considers both the physical and psychological impact. Therapy, mindfulness, physical activity, and social support can help reset the body's stress response. For recovery, understanding and addressing trauma's wide-ranging effects on the body is key, emphasizing how the mind and body are interconnected.

The Nervous System's Role

When you're traumatized, your nervous system plays a huge role. Basically, it's the body's communication system, sending, receiving, and interpreting information. There are two parts to the nervous system: the central nervous system, which is the brain and spinal cord, and the peripheral nervous system, which is all the rest of the nerves and sensory cells. In times of trauma, the nervous system coordinates the body's immediate reactions. This involves activating the sympathetic nervous system, a part of the peripheral nervous system that controls fight or flight. As a result of this activation, stress hormones are released, the heart rate increases, breathing speeds up, and muscles get ready for action. It should be noted, however, that the nervous system's response to trauma extends far beyond this initial response. Chronic or unresolved trauma can cause regulatory chaos in the sympathetic nervous system and parasympathetic nervous system. In a perfect world, both nervous systems would be in balance: the sympathetic nervous system mobilizes the body's resources when under stress, while the parasympathetic nervous system promotes digestion and rest. Trauma can lead to an imbalance though, leading to an overactive sympathetic nervous system and an underactive parasympathetic

29

nervous system. As the body is on high alert all the time, this imbalance can lead to chronic stress, anxiety, and other health problems.

Additionally, trauma can affect the central nervous system, especially the brain. This can affect your amygdala (which processes emotions) your hippocampus (which regulates stress and memory), and your prefrontal cortex (which handles decisions and impulses). These changes can make it hard to control your emotions, remember things, and make good decisions.

Treatments for trauma often involve strategies aimed at helping the body restore balance and regulating its nervous system's response to stress, which is key to developing effective treatments You can do this with therapeutic techniques, mindfulness practices, and other interventions.

Embedded trauma and its release

An embedded trauma is when a traumatic experience is deeply ingrained in an individual's psyche and body. When it comes to embedded trauma, unlike memories, it sticks around, manifesting itself in different ways in the form of physical, emotional, or psychological symptoms. It can cause chronic pain, anxiety, depression, flashbacks, and a general feeling of unease. It's embedded because it hasn't been adequately addressed or processed, causing the body and mind to continue acting like it's still happening. Healing embedded trauma involves both a mind-body approach. Since the nervous system plays a big role in trauma response, treatment often focuses on calming you down. Getting out of the fight-or-flight state allows the nervous system to recalibrate. Therapies like somatic experiencing can help you become more aware of your body and release tension.

In a safe environment, trauma-focused therapies like EMDR (Eye Movement Desensitization and Reprocessing) can help people reprocess traumatic memories, so they don't feel so intrusive and overwhelming. Meditation and mindfulness can also

31

help people become more present and less distracted by traumatic memories or anxiety. Body-based practices like yoga, tai chi, or qigong can help you release trauma by enhancing a deeper mind-body connection, reducing stress, and promoting relaxation. If you can't find the words to express your emotions, music and art therapy can help. There's usually a gradual release of trauma, which requires patience, self-compassion, and support. Creating a new narrative and body memory that doesn't revolve around the trauma allows you to move on with a better sense of freedom.

Releasing Trauma from the Body

To release trauma from the body, we must understand that trauma can manifest physically as well as emotionally or psychologically. Release of trauma begins with recognizing its physical signs, like chronic tension or altered breathing.

For this process to work, you need to create a sense of safety. You can do this by setting up a supportive environment and using grounding techniques. By guiding attention to body sensations linked to trauma, somatic therapies can be profoundly trans-formative for healing.

The practice of mindfulness and meditation helps you connect with the present moment and observe body sensations without reacting, helping you deal with trauma related emotions. Incorporating physical movement can also help since it lets you release tension and stress in your body.

Building a Foundation for Healing

During times of significant stress, laying a solid foundation is like building a house, where safety and stability are essential. To start, we've got to give yourself a sense of safety, which might take different forms depending on your needs. Some might get it from physical space, others might get it from emotional support.

Being kind to yourself is essential to this process, as well as accepting that healing is a journey full of complexities. It's also important to set healthy boundaries as well. It's about figuring out what's acceptable in how people treat you and how you treat yourself.

I can't stress enough how important it is to have a support system - friends, family, and professionals who are there to offer comfort and guidance when things get tough. Additionally, mind-body practices like mindfulness and yoga help bridge the gap between mental and physical health, grounding you in the present and reducing stress.

Healing can be done through reflection, whether that's through journaling, therapy, or meditation. Fitness, sleep, and nutrition are also key pieces of this foundation - they not only support physical well-being but also help you cope with stress. Finally, adopting a growth mindset reframes healing as an opportunity to transform obstacles into lessons and promote a sense of hope.

Part 3

Think about standing at the edge of a serene lake, the surface a perfect mirror, reflecting the sky, the trees, and the very essence of the world around you. Now that you're aware and clear, you're taking the first step to healing. The idea is to look inward, get to know your own experiences, emotions, and body sensations, and recognize their reflections. Getting in touch with this inner clarity is the first step on a transformative path, turning obstacles into stepping stones and shadows into areas just begging for illumination.

THE ROLE OF AWARENESS IN HEALING

Awareness plays a big role in healing, acting as a foundation for recovery and wellbeing. Awareness is about acknowledging and understanding one's feelings, thoughts, bodily sensations, and behaviors. It's important for a lot of reasons.

Firstly, awareness lets you see what's hidden, especially traumatized experiences. By noticing our internal states, we can identify patterns that might be causing us pain, like negative thought loops, suppressed feelings, or harmful coping mechanisms.

35

First step to change is to acknowledge, as we can't heal what we don't acknowledge.

Awareness enhances a deeper connection with the self. It promotes a compassionate, non-judgmental dialogue within, where feelings and thoughts can be observed. A key to healing is self-compassion, as it shifts the inner narrative from one of shame and self-blame to one of kindness and understanding.

As well as being aware of our well-being within ourselves, awareness extends to our relationships, environments, and social dynamics. The more we understand how these external conditions impact our mental and emotional health, the more informed our choices will be.

As part of the therapeutic process, awareness helps you explore and understand. You'll learn how to unravel complicated emotions and uncover limiting beliefs in therapy. Awareness leads to growth when guided by a therapist.

Finally, awareness helps you be present. A lot of healing challenges come from dwelling on past hurts or fearing the future. Being present allows you to break free from the shackles of the past and future, engaging with life more openly and curiously. In summary, awareness is crucial to healing. Through it, we're able to illuminate the unseen, nurture self-compassion, connect our minds and bodies, make better choices, provide therapeutic insight, and stay present. Healing becomes more accessible and empowered when people see healing through the lens of awareness.

A sense of being in tune with your body, often called somatic awareness, is when you're aware of your own physical sensations, needs, and reactions. A dynamic dialogue between your mind and body can promote health, well-being, and personal growth. You notice your body's subtle cues when you're tuned in. They range from hunger and fatigue to tension and relaxation in different parts of the body.

Recognizing how your emotions manifest physically can help you deal with them, whether it's a shortened heartbeat when you're anxious or a heaviness in your limbs when you're sad. By practicing self-care and health-promoting behaviors, you'll be better off physically and mentally.

Emotional regulation is also enhanced by being in tune with your body. It's easier to deal with your emotional needs if you understand how your feelings affect your body. For example, you might notice that certain situations cause a knot in your stomach, signaling anxiety or fear. It's easier to deal with the underlying emotions if you know what's going on with your body.

Reduced stress and anxiety can also be achieved through body awareness. Stress can be managed through relaxation techniques, exercise, or other coping mechanisms if you detect it early. Preventing stress from building up and having a negative impact on your health is key.

Getting in tune with your body isn't just about noticing discomfort or stress; it's also about recognizing pleasure, relaxation, and well-being. Having this positive awareness can make you more likely to do things that make you happy and fulfilled.

Body awareness can be developed through practices like mindfulness meditation, yoga, tai chi, or just checking in with your body throughout the day. With time, these practices can help you build a more harmonious and balanced relationship with your body.

The Healing Power of Presence

It's all about being versus doing. Healing isn't just about doing, it's also about being. Being present with one's experiences without judgment is the key to enjoying them. With grounding techniques, you can reduce feelings of overwhelm and disconnect often associated with trauma by anchoring yourself to the present moment.

Incorporating awareness practices into daily routines, makes mundane activities turn into opportunities for mindfulness. Routine is key here. Set up a routine of self-awareness practices to support healing. You've got to build a compassion relationship with yourself. Self-compassion plays a crucial role in healing, and by adopting strategies that promote kind words and forgiveness toward oneself, you can enhance healing.

It's like learning to navigate by the stars. It's like having a guiding light to help us navigate our inner worlds. You can experience profound healing and transformation when you become more attuned to your inner self. Remember, self-awareness isn't a destination. It's a pathway to a deeper, more reso-nant connection with yourself and with the world.

CHAPTER 2

Part 1

BEGINNING YOUR SOMATIC JOURNEY

Think about the symphony of emotions you're experiencing every moment. There's so much information in your body, from the rhythmic cadence of your heartbeat to the gentle rise and fall of your breath. You'll be able to tune in and listen to your body's unique signal once you take your first steps on your somatic journey. When you turn the dial on a radio, you find a clear signal; The goal of this chapter is to help you listen to your body Starting with Self-Awareness.

Being aware of your own body is like learning a new language. By listening to your body, you'll understand its needs, discomforts, and joys. In short, awareness is the very first and most important step toward healing, resilience, and forming a profound connection with oneself.

Start by practicing exercises designed to sharpen your body's signals and perception. You can begin by sitting quietly for a few minutes, where you may close your eyes and turn your attention inward. Feel what's going on without judgment: What sensations are there? Where do you feel tension, and where do you feel ease? By practicing deep listening, we establish a responsive relationship with our bodies rather than a reactive one.

What is a responsive and reactive relationship, and their difference?

A responsive relationship in your body means it can adapt to changes in a balanced and proactive way, ensuring smooth, regulated function. As an example, adjusting hormone levels or preparing immunity for changes.

A reactive relationship involves immediate, often short-term responses to stimuli, like sudden fires of adrenaline or inflammation after an injury. Despite being crucial for immediate defense or healing, excessive reactivity without balance can be stressful.

Guided body scans are another great way to get in touch with yourself. From your toes to your crown, systematically pay attention to different parts of your body as you lie down or sit. Take a moment to notice the sensations in each area - warmth, coolness, tingling, tightness, and acknowledge them gently. Exercises like this improve your sensory vocabulary and make you more aware of your body.

Following a foundation of stillness and scanning, we explore how your body communicates through movement. You can learn how different parts of your body feel when you slowly lift and lower your arms or turn your head side-to-side. What do your joints feel like? Can you tell me where there's fluidity and where there's resistance? The practice helps you understand how emotions manifest physically and how movement can ease stress.

It's important to listen to your body if you feel resistance in movement. Don't push yourself through pain or discomfort. Adjust your movements, do gentle stretching or strengthening exercises, and if the resistance persists, talk to a doctor.

Bringing self-awareness to your day turns routine actions into somatic exploration. If you're walking, cooking, or doing anything else, periodically check in with your body. How do you feel? Is there anything you can do to make moving easier and less stressful? By checking in on-the-go, you reinforce the habit of mindful presence and self-care.

As you begin your somatic journey, you're acknowledging your body's wisdom and telling your story. From here on out, you'll begin a journey of increased self-awareness, understanding, and compassion. Using your body's signals will not only make you more present, but it will also open a direct channel to your inner world, where healing and insight await. Here's to a transformative adventure - let's get curious and open-hearted.

Part 2

Picture this: When life gets crazy, with its deadlines, demands, and constant digital chatter, there's a simple, powerful tool that can bring you balance and tranquility. There are no batteries, wireless, or special equipment required for this tool. It's as natural as living. It's your breath. The key to stress relief and emotional regulation is breathing. You don't even think about it, but it's so important. Let's explore the basics of breathing, uncovering simple techniques that can transform turbulence into calm and chaos into tranquility

BREATH WORK BASICS

Although our breath is our constant companion, it has the potential to heal and transform. Bringing conscious awareness to our breathing can help us manage stress and anxiety and enhance our sense of well-being.

Our first step is to look at breath work's physiological impact, understanding how it can affect our nervous system, reduce cortisol levels, and improve overall health. In this section, we demystify the science behind breathwork, making it a lot more relatable and accessible. Following that, we introduce several breathing techniques with step-by-step instructions.

The practice of breath-work improves wellbeing by acting on the nervous system, reducing stress hormones like cortisol, and improving overall health. Taking deep, slow breaths activate our parasympathetic nervous system, which calms our bodies, lowers our blood pressure, and moves us from our stress-induced "fight or flight" response to a relaxed "rest and digest" state. By lowering cortisol levels, chronic stress conditions like insomnia and anxiety can be mitigated.

Breathing exercises also improve circulation and oxygen exchange, boosting mental and physical energy. It's also good for your emotional health, alleviating anxiety and depression symptoms, and keeping you calm and focused. In essence, breath-work helps manage stress, improve physiological function, and enhance mental and emotional well-being, so it's important to maintain balance and health. Deep Abdominal Breathing - Engage your diaphragm fully to breathe deeper, more soothingly for better relaxation.

Make yourself comfortable. Sit or lie down.

One hand on the chest, one on the belly.

Deeply inhale through your nose, letting your belly rise more than your chest.

Feel your belly and chest drop as you exhale slowly.

For several minutes, focus on slow, deep breaths.

The 4-7-8 Technique - Here's a simple and powerful method to calm your mind and prepare your body for sleep, ideal for moments of anxiety.

Let's inhale for 4 seconds through our noses.

For 7 seconds, hold your breath.

For 8 seconds, exhale fully through your mouth.

You can repeat as many times as you want.

Equal Breathing - Harmonize your inhalations and exhalations to enhance emotional balance and focus.

Count to 4 while you inhale through your nose.

Count to 4 while you exhale through your nose.

Aim to get equal inhales and exhales and adjust seconds if necessary.

Breath work can enhance your everyday life if you incorporate these practices into your routine.

No matter where you are, whether you're at work, sitting in traffic, or exercising,

you can practice mindful breathing. This is going to help you grow and take care of yourself.

Part 3

When we're rushing around and time is a luxury, imagine having a secret sanctuary of calm, an invisible sanctuary where peace is just a breath away. There is no fantasy in this, but it is a reality that can be achieved by practicing the simple, powerful breathing technique we mentioned previously, called deep abdominal breathing. You're not just taking deep breaths; you're transforming stress into serenity, putting an end to agitation, right there, wherever you are, whatever you're doing. Here are three more easy, on-the-go breathing exercises you can add to your busy schedule to stay calm at any time.

THREE ON-THE-GO EXERCISES FOR BREATHING

1. The Traffic Light Breath

When to use it - Waiting at a traffic light or in transit.

How to do it - Put one hand on your belly. Slowly inhale through your nose, feeling your hand rise in response. At the top of your inhale, pause, then slowly exhale through your mouth, feeling your hand drop. Repeat this breathing pattern until the light changes or your stop arrives.

Benefits - Focus on calm and control, and you'll turn a usually stressful pause into an opportunity for re-juvenation.

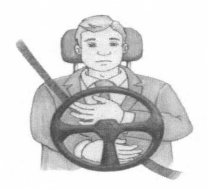

2. The lift (or elevator) Breather

When to use it - Riding a lift or waiting for one.

How to do it - Hands by your side, feet slightly apart. Let your breath move with the lift as it climbs or descends. When the lift goes up, inhale slowly and deeply. Pause for a moment when it stops. Then exhale slowly as it goes down. You don't have to be in a lift to imagine one.

Benefits - By anchoring yourself in the present moment, you reduce anxiety and hurry, and you transform a mundane activity into something calming and centered.

3. The Walking Breath

When to use it - Walking to your next appointment, class, or errand.

How to do it - Your breathing and walking pace should be your focus. Breathe in for four steps, hold your breath for two, and then exhale for four steps. Depending on your walking speed and comfort level, adjust the counts.

Benefits - It combines breathwork with movement, promoting mindfulness and a sense of calm. As well as improving coordination, this exercise improves breathing rhythm.

Using these exercises, you can turn idle or transitional moments into mindfulness and stress relief. It is your secret weapon, your tool that you use to combat the chaos of the day and is always on hand to use when you need them. If you incorporate these on-the go breathing exercises into your daily routine, you'll develop a habit of mindfulness that can dramatically improve your health. It is with great pleasure that I welcome you to the journey of integrating deep, abdominal breathing into the fabric of your life - where calm is always just a breath away.

CHAPTER 3

Part 1

THE SCIENCE OF STRESS AND YOUR BODY

If you were to imagine for a moment you were walking through a dense forest, and suddenly, from behind, the sounds of rustling leaves and breaking twigs were heard. As a result, your heart rates increase, your breath quickens, and your muscles tense in a fraction of a second, before you have a chance to think about the potential danger, your body goes into automatic alarm mode. There is no better way to describe this instantaneous change in your body than the stress response, which is your body's ancient and primal response to perceived threats.

The Stress Response

Stress response is at the heart of our survival mechanism, a complex system designed to keep us safe. A series of physiological changes prepare our bodies to take on challenges.

We can become chronically stressed when the pressure of modern life constantly activates this system, affecting our happiness, health, and quality of life.

When we feel threatened, our body undergoes an immediate transformation, controlled by the sympathetic nervous system. We are primed for action by hormones like adrenaline and cortisol, which increase heart rate, blood pressure, and glucose levels. In the presence of genuine danger, this response is invaluable, but it can wear and tear your body and mind with frequent activation.

The stress response is triggered not just by external events, but by our perception of them. Realizing this opens a lot of possibilities. With tools like the somatic practices and mindfulness techniques found in this book, we can change how we perceive stress, reducing its effects.

Knowing how the stress response works will make it easier to apply the somatic exercises in this book and mitigate stress. Pendulation, segmenting, and mindful movement, which we will discuss later, become much more than exercises in body awareness, and they help us to overcome stress and handle life's challenges more effectively.

During our exploration of how stress affects the body, we also discover the profound power of somatic practices to transform our relationship with stress. We can live a more balanced, healthier life when we learn how to modulate our response to our body's signals.

So how does stress affect us? Our bodies, minds, and behaviors are all affected by stress. As soon as we experience stress, our bodies begin to move into action, initiating a series of changes within us that can be detrimental to our well-being. Our heart beats faster, our muscles tense up, and we might feel sick. If stress persists, it can cause heart disease, weakened immunity, and digestive problems.

Mentally, stress can be a double-edged sword. Initially, it might heighten our senses and sharpen our focus to deal with immediate challenges. However, chronic stress wears down our mental resilience, leading to irritability, anxiety, depression, and difficulties with concentration and memory. These mental and emotional strains can affect our behavior, disrupting sleep, changing our eating habits, and possibly leading us to rely on substances like alcohol or drugs for relief. It should also be noted that stress often causes us to withdraw from social interactions, which isolates us at a time when we need support the most.

The cycle of stress affecting our physical health can further amplify our mental stress, creating a loop that's challenging to break. By understanding the comprehensive impact of stress, we can develop strategies that address both our physical and mental well-being, such as regular exercise, mindfulness, relaxation, and nurturing supportive relationships.

It's not just about why deep abdominal breathing, Qigong, and EFT tapping work, but also about how to use these techniques when we need them most (we'll talk about Qigong in chapter 5 and EFT tapping in chapter 6). As we continue our somatic journey, let this knowledge be a foundation upon which we build a deeper, more harmonious connection between mind, body, and the environment around us, turning the science of stress into a pathway for personal transformation and healing.

The stress response is not an enemy, it's a built-in survival mechanism that has served humans throughout history. We live in a world where stress is rarely life-threatening, but our bodies act like it is. When we understand the science behind the stress response, we can start taking control. By understanding stress, we can manage it better, leading to a healthier, happier life. You've made it to the beginning of your journey to mastering your stress response.

Part 2

How do some people bounce back from stressful situations so much faster than others? How do some people stay calm when they're under pressure?

There lies the secret to how this is possible, and it lies within the incredible concepts of neuroplasticity and neuro regeneration resilience. The experiences, thoughts, and actions around you constantly shape and reshape your brain. The key to breaking the stress cycle is flexibility. By understanding neuroplasticity and resilience, you can turn overwhelming waves into manageable ripples.

BREAKING THE STRESS CYCLE

What is neuroplasticity? Neuroplasticity is your brain's ability to reorganize itself in response to new experiences, learning, or injury. Our brains aren't fixed, they can change over time. We shape our neural pathways by repeated experiences and thoughts. **Keeping your brain fit** - You can promote positive brain change with positive affirmations, meditation, cognitive-behavioral strategies, and mindfulness. Those can help rewire our brains so they're less stressed.

58

Resilience in a person: What it is - When someone is resilient, they can deal with problems mentally or emotionally in a crisis and return to pre-crisis status quickly and can cope with adversity without enduring any long-term negative consequences. In managing stress, this is key.

The building blocks of resilience - Some of these are self-awareness, mindfulness, selfcare, positive relationships, flexibility, and optimism. These practical strategies will help you break the stress cycle.

Practicing mindfulness - Mindfulness exercises that are easy to incorporate into your day-to-day. They can help you relax and stay in the moment.

Cognitive Techniques - Using cognitive techniques to change stress-inducing thoughts. You can reduce anxiety and stress by changing your negative thinking.

Habits That Work - Lifestyle factors, like sleep, nutrition, and physical activity, play a big role in stress management. You can reduce your stress levels by making little changes in your life.

Set boundaries and manage your time - It's important to set healthy boundaries and manage your time to reduce stress and mental health problems.

We can change our relationship with stress with neuroplasticity and resilience. We can reduce stress in our daily lives with several on-the-go practices that I'm about to show you. You're getting stronger and more adaptable with every step you take. Prepare to shape your mind with openness and curiosity.

Part 3

The hustle and bustle of day-to-day life can lead to stress building up until our shoulders feel like they're carrying the weight of the world, and our necks feel stiff as they brace against the wind. You might be surprised to hear that relief could be just a few simple movements away, no matter where you are. As a secret weapon, these on the-go exercises can help you dispel stress and tension with ease and effectiveness, transforming any moment into a time of relaxation and release, no matter where you are in the world.

THREE ON-THE-GO EXERCISES FOR TENSION RELIEF

1. Taking care of business shoulder rolls

When to use it - This is perfect for when you're waiting in line, sitting in traffic, or taking a short break. This is an effective way for you to relax your muscles and can be repeated several times throughout the day as a means of easing tension.

How to do It - It is important that you stand or sit with your back straight. Make circles with your shoulders by lifting them toward your ears, then rolling them back. Inhale as you lift your shoulders, then exhale as you roll them back. Ten rolls, then 10 in the other direction.

Benefits - It helps release tension in the shoulder and neck area, where stress often accumulates. Exercise increases blood flow and releases endorphins, reducing stress naturally.

2. Releasing the Pressure neck stretches

When to use it - Ideal for a quick break while working on the computer, after a phone call, or even while travelling. Several times a day will keep neck stiffness away.

How to do It - Make sure your spine is straight when you sit or stand. Take a deep breath and tilt your head towards one shoulder until you feel a gentle stretch on the opposite side of your neck. Breathe deeply whilst doing this and hold this position for 15-30 seconds, then gently lift your head back to the center and repeat on the other side.

Benefits - Having tight neck tension in your muscles can cause headaches and stress. Relaxing neck

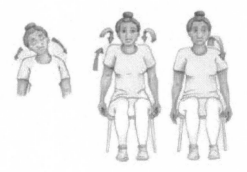

stretches relieve tension, improve mobility, and re-duce stress.

3. Unwinding the Strain with wrist and hand Stretches

When to use it - If you're reading emails, writing or typing, or even scrolling through your phone, this is ideal. It's easy to do and can easily be incorporated into your day for regular stress relief.

How to do It - Stretch one arm out in front of you, palm facing up. Then gently press down on the out-stretched hand's fingers with the other hand, stretch-ing the forearm and wrist. You hold for 15-30 sec-onds, then switch hands. In the next step, make a fist and then fan your fingers as wide as you can, mak-ing sure you stretch them as much as possible. You should repeat this step 5-10 times for each hand.

Benefits - Most of us spend hours typing or on our phones, which leads to wrist and hand tension. You can prevent strain and reduce stress by stretching these areas.

Stress levels and overall well-being can be improved significantly by incorporating these simple, effective exercises into your daily life. With their ease of use, they help you tackle stress anywhere, anytime. When you take the time to focus on your body and release tension, you will find that you will be able to refresh your mind, lighten your load, and approach your daily tasks with renewed calm and focus that will make you more effective and efficient. Enjoy these on-the-go exercises as your ally for getting through the day.

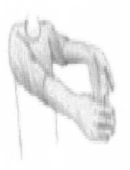 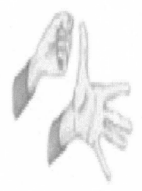

CHAPTER 4
PART 1

HEALING TRAUMA THROUGH THE BODY

Imagine taking on a journey through peaks and valleys, learning to navigate the terrain so you can heal yourself. In somatic therapy, pendulation and titration are powerful techniques that can help you heal trauma through your body in a gentle, yet profound way. The goal of these methods is to move through past pain with awareness, care, and gradual engagement. With the help of these techniques, we can learn how to process trauma in a way that respects our bodies' natural rhythm and healing capacity.

PENDULATION AND TITRATION
Pendulation

Pendulation is a body-focused therapy developed by Dr. Peter A. Levine. Stress and trauma can be healed with this method. When we talk about pendulation, it's the natural rhythm between states of contraction and expansion, or between sensations of discomfort and comfort. Based on the observation that, in nature, animals oscillate between states of arousal and relaxation following a threatening event, which helps them discharge the energy associated with it and return to balance. The symptoms of trauma can become stuck in our bodies because of suppressing natural oscillations due to societal norms, religious or personal beliefs, or a lack of safe opportunities.

Therapy helps you notice sensations, emotions, and images, and helps you pendulate between activating (distressing) and deactivating (comforting) experiences. By doing this, you can safely experience and integrate overwhelming feelings and sensations, thereby releasing traumatic stress.

By encouraging the natural ebb and flow of physiological and emotional states, pendulation in somatic experience helps the nervous system regain its self-regulation abilities. As a result, you'll be more resilient, able to handle stress and feel more balanced and happier.

66

How to practice Pendulation

These are the steps you can take on your own to practice pendulation, especially if you're dealing with stress or mild discomfort (not severe trauma, which should be handled by a therapist):

Find a comfortable spot. Put yourself in a quiet, safe place where you won't be interrupted.

Get your feet on the ground - Take a deep breath and ground yourself. You can do this by noticing the sensations in your feet, focusing on your breath, or feeling the chair or floor.

Identify sensations - Be aware of any sensations in your body. Try to identify one area where you feel tension or discomfort and one area where you feel more relaxed.

Let's focus on discomfort - Take a moment to focus on the discomfort. Feel any sensations, feelings, or thoughts here. You don't have to push yourself into pain or stress, just notice what's going on.

Comfort mode - Put your attention on the area of your body that feels comfortable or neutral. Allow yourself to relax into these sensations.

Pendulate - Gently switch between the uncomfortable and comfortable sensations. Switch back and forth between the two sides.

Observe the changes - Pay attention to your emotions and sensations as you pendulate. In this exercise, you will observe if your ability to feel comfortable has increased or if the areas of discomfort have become less intense.

Finished with comfort - Be sure to end the session by focusing on the comfortable or neutral sensations.

Reflection - Reflect on your experience afterwards. If you are experiencing any physical or emotional changes, please note them.

It's not about getting rid of discomfort; In fact, it's all about improving the way the body manages your senses, so you can experience a better life. You should stop and consider seeing a therapist if this

practice triggers significant emotional distress, especially if you're suffering from deep-seated trauma
or severe anxiety.

Titration

It's important to understand that titration helps people cope with trauma without feeling overwhelmed.
By working with physical sensations and emotions
gently and gradually, you won't overwhelm the
nervous system. By slowly introducing small, manageable amounts of traumatic material or intense
emotions, you can process and integrate these experiences. If these steps aren't overdone, they prevent
traumatization and support the body's natural healing mechanisms. The benefits of titration include
being able to increase your tolerance of difficult
emotions and sensations safely and effectively,
which promotes emotional resilience and recovery.

How to practice Titration

Practicing titration on your own should be done
with caution. Start with mild stress, make sure
you've got coping strategies, and don't dive into

traumatic material without professional help. You don't want to push through or relive traumatic experiences; you want to nurture a sense of safety and control. Stop practicing if you're feeling overwhelmed and get help.

Establish a safe environment - It's important to build trust and safety before starting trauma work. Make sure there are coping strategies and support systems in place. This is done by slowly experiencing challenging emotions and sensations in small, manageable increments to build tolerance and aid healing without causing distress.

A grounding technique - This can include mindfulness practices, deep breathing, or focusing on physical sensations like touching a piece of fabric or holding a cold object.

Identify trauma memories - The first step towards healing is identifying specific traumatic memories or triggers. As with any kind of therapy, the first step is often to work on less distressing memories, and then gradually move on to the more troubling ones.

Tolerances - Be aware of your tolerance and emotional reaction all the time. Make sure you're watching your reactions. Engage with the traumatic memory without getting overwhelmed.

Exposure must be gradual - Don't overload yourself with the traumatic memory; start slow. Writing, storytelling, and visualization are all great ways to do this.

Process - Process your thoughts and feelings about the trauma. You can work through your emotions and beliefs that arise.

Regulation - The therapist (if you are using one) will help regulate your emotions during and after exposure. Use coping strategies to manage distress or go back to grounding.

Reflect on it - Whenever you finish a session, think about it. Having a trusted friend or therapist who understands what was learned, how you coped, and a plan for the future is helpful.

Maintaining your health and well-being - Taking care of yourself outside of therapy and utilizing friends and family. Recovery depends on it.

You may wish to consider seeking specialized training in trauma-informed care if you are interested in practicing this technique as a therapist. A trauma survivor should work with a therapist who understands how to navigate trauma therapy safely.

Titration is, in essence, a method of working through traumatic experiences in a safe, controlled, and manageable manner, allowing the individual to be able to heal without being overwhelmed by their experiences during trauma therapy. A compassionate, paced approach to trauma healing can be achieved by introducing pendulation and titration. By respecting the wisdom of the body and its inherent ability to heal, these techniques help you navigate trauma without becoming overwhelmed. These pages are your invitation to embrace the gentle undulations of healing, and learn to move through trauma with grace, understanding, and renewed energy.

How to combine Pendulation and Titration

When pendulation and titration are combined in therapy, it's a step-by-step approach that helps people through traumatic experiences.

Ensure safety and grounding - Create a safe, supportive environment. Make sure you're emotionally and physically stable by using grounding techniques.

Find a resource - Those memories, thoughts, or sensations that make you feel safe, comfortable, or happy. In the process, we'll use these resources to return to feeling safe.

Titration first - Choose a small, manageable piece (a memory, feeling, or sensation) from the traumatic experience. Make sure it's something you can handle.

Now you pendulate- Put your focus on the chosen element of trauma (the titrated element). Keep an eye on your response to make sure it's within your tolerance.

Move to a resource - Put your focus on the pre-iden-tified resource before you get overwhelmed. Take advantage of the safety and comfort it offers.

Pendulate Between Sensations - Bring yourself back to the traumatic element, then back to the re-source. Always remember to move between these two points so you don't get overwhelmed.

Keeping an eye on things - Keep an eye on your re-actions and adjust the intensity and pace accord-ingly. Making sure the process is therapeutic and manageable is key.

Process and Integrate - Allow yourself time to pro-cess and discuss new feelings or insights. Together, you'll be able to see things differently.

Increasing gradually - Slowly increase the intensity or duration of the traumatic exposure as you get more comfortable.

Shutting down the session - Finish each session by making sure the person feels safe and grounded. Look at how the session went and what you learned. A continual support system - Support and encouragement will come from a therapist or trusted friend. You can adjust the approach based on your needs.

It's important to remember that pendulation and titration are delicate processes that should be guided by a trained therapist, especially when it comes to trauma. This controlled and supportive approach builds resilience and enhances emotional regulation.

Part 2

When we're healing, it's like discovering a hidden treasure. A place of safety within, is crucial for healing trauma. This is about creating a safe space for us to be seen, heard, and protected, so we can approach trauma work not as a battle, but as a healing process. By examining what it means to feel safe inside yourself and why it's the backbone of trauma recovery, we can transform our inner landscape into a place of strength and calm. The purpose of this section is to explain the difference between external and internal safety.

SAFE SPACES WITHIN THE SELF

External safety refers to the physical safety of an environment. There's no threat or harm from outside sources, like other people or things. This includes safe living spaces, safe communities, and protection from violence.

On the other hand, internal safety is about feeling secure emotionally or psychologically. Feeling safe in yourself includes feeling stable, grounded, and secure in your feelings and thoughts. In other words, it involves managing stress, regulating emotions, and having a strong sense of self. The key elements required to establish a sense of safety within, include self-awareness, self-compassion, and grounding techniques.

Building Your Internal Sanctuary

First, create a safe, comforting space in your imagination. Choose a quiet spot and sit or lie comfortably. Close your eyes and breathe deeply and relax your body. Get a sense of your safe space. Imagine yourself in a place that makes you feel safe and happy. It doesn't matter whether it's real or not. Make it vivid by adding details. Not only include what you see in your mind's eye but also what you hear, feel, smell, and taste. Feel safe by including comforting items. Use a physical gesture to convey this calm feeling. Be sure to visit your safe space often to strengthen its presence.

In trauma work, we need self-compassion. Be kind to yourself, especially when you're facing painful memories or feelings. Set and maintain healthy boundaries with others and within yourself. To set boundaries in yourself, you need to define your values, limits, and acceptable behaviors, then commit to upholding these standards. To set boundaries with others, you need to communicate your limits, needs, and expectations, and consistently enforce them. Creating safe spaces within us gives us the courage and grace we need to confront trauma. It's all about creating and maintaining these internal sanctuaries, so you can take care of yourself and take steps toward healing.

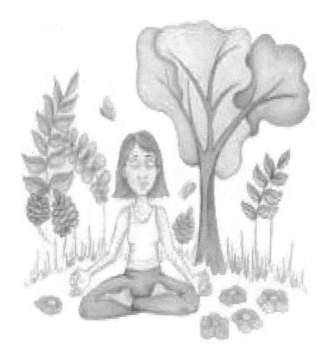

Part 3

When people are working through trauma, pendulation and titration are best done by a trained professional. However, it's possible to practice gentle, adapted exercises inspired by these on-the-go techniques to reduce stress and regulate emotions. You can do these exercises to manage stress without getting into deep trauma.

THREE ON-THE-GO EXERCISES FOR PENDULA-TION AND TITRATION

1. Breath Awareness Pendulation

When to use it - It can be used during stressful moments, when feeling anxious, when transitioning between different activities, or to ground yourself when you feel overwhelmed. The techniques are portable tools to help you manage stress and boost mindfulness.

How to do it -

Find - Feel something neutral or slightly pleasant in your body (e.g., warmth in your hands, grass under your feet).

Focus - Be aware of the sensation's qualities (temperature, texture, weight) for a moment.

Shift - Put your focus on your breath. Keep an eye on your inhalation and exhalation rhythms without changing them.

Alternate - Once you have breathed for a few breaths, try focusing your attention back on something pleasant or neutral, and then every few breaths switch your focus between your breath and this sensation.

Reflect - Finish by noticing how your body feels. Don't forget that the goal isn't to remove stress, but to notice and appreciate how your body feels.

Benefits - An improved sense of calm and bodily awareness, reduced stress and anxiety, and improved focus.

2. Grounding Titration

When to use it - While engaging in everyday activities, to help you get back to a calm and balanced state when you're feeling overwhelmed, triggered, or disoriented.

How to do it -

Ground - Keep your feet on the ground. Get a feel for the floor beneath you.

Notice - Recall a mild stressor (something that was annoying but not too bad). Observe where you feel it.

Return - Refocus on your feet, feeling grounded and supported by the ground.

Alternate - Your attention should alternate between the mild stressor and the ground beneath your feet. Focus more on grounding than the stressor.

Reflect – Finish by keeping your attention on your feet and noticing anything that changes.

Benefits - The ability to handle and recover from emotional triggers and overwhelming situations with a reduced level of anxiety and stress.

3. Sensory Pendulation

When to use it - It's great for stress management, switching between tasks, emotional balance, and re-gaining awareness of your body.

How to do it -

Observe - Look at something you find pleasant or neutral (nature, sky, art).

Engage - Observe the colors, shapes, and textures of this object. When you look at the object, pay attention to any pleasant feelings or emotions you have.

Switch - Give yourself a minute to think about something mildly stressful. Observe where this feels in your body.

Return - Take your attention back to the pleasant or neutral object, immerse yourself in the observation, and allow your senses to be overwhelmed by the sensation that comes along with it.

Balance - You should continue to gently pendulate between the stressor and the object, making sure that you spend more time with the object. You should always end on the positive side of things; in this case, it is the object.

Benefits - Improved emotional regulation, more resilience to stress, improved body awareness, and staying grounded and present during challenging or overwhelming times.

Remember, these are stress management exercises, not deep trauma therapy. The exercises should only be practiced with mild stressors to get the best results. If you are experiencing intense emotions or physical sensations, a good suggestion would be to pause and ground yourself in the present moment. You might find it beneficial to talk to a mental

health professional if these exercises trigger you or
overwhelm you.

CHAPTER 5

Part 1

INTEGRATING MIND AND BODY WITH QIGONG

Imagine discovering a practice that harmonizes your body and mind and connects you to a centuries-old healing tradition. Qigong is an ancient Chinese practice that combines gentle movement, deep breathing, and meditation to promote harmony, health, and vitality. With roots in Taoist, Buddhist, and martial arts traditions, Qigong isn't just a workout; it's a way to enhance well-being, a way to connect the physical and the spiritual, and a way to find peace within.

Introduction to Qigong

Known as "chee-gung," qigong is a centuries-old system of body posture, movement, breathing, and meditation used for health, spirituality, and martial arts training.

Originally from Chinese culture, it's part of Traditional Chinese Medicine (TCM). 'Qigong' comes from 'Qi' (life energy) and 'Gong' (a skill developed by steady practice). The practices of qigong can be categorized in various ways, but most commonly they are divided into two categories:

Qigong that's dynamic or active (Dong Gong). It involves breathing and postures coordinated with mental focus. It helps develop and balance your Qi. Movements can improve your health or address specific health problems.

Qigong that is static or passive. It's all about meditative poses, breathing techniques, and internal stillness, with lots of meditation. A big goal of this form is to develop mental peace, deep inner awareness, and a sense of connection with the universe.

The practice of Qigong is said to boost health and vitality by balancing and harnessing the body's Qi. Not only does it help you with your physical health, but it helps with your mental health as well, like stress reduction and concentration. Each style and tradition of qigong has its own set of practices and theories. The most popular forms are Tai Chi, Ba

86

Duan Jin, and Yi Jin Jing. Although Qigong is rooted in Chinese medicine and philosophy, it's now practiced by people all over the world. It's gentle practice that anyone can do, no matter what their fitness level is. As with any physical or meditative practice, learning Qigong from an instructor ensures your techniques are performed correctly.

The Multifaceted Benefits of Qigong

Qigong has a lot of benefits for physical, mental, and emotional health. A regular Qigong practice can do a lot for you like

Improved Physical Health. The exercises in Qigong can improve your strength, flexibility, balance, and stamina. It helps with cardiovascular, respiratory, circulatory, lymphatic, and digestive problems. It can help manage or alleviate symptoms of chronic illnesses like hypertension, heart disease, cancer, arthritis, fibromyalgia, and chronic fatigue.

Reducing stress. You can reduce stress, anxiety, and depression with Qigong's gentle, rhythmic movements. Stress hormones are reduced when the mind

87

is calmed. This promotes a feeling of well-being, and your sleep patterns can improve.

Increased mental focus and clarity. Regular Qigong practice can help you concentrate, remember, and make better decisions. By meditating, you'll clear your mind, reduce mental clutter, and feel more alert.

Balanced Energy Levels. With Qigong, you'll get more vitality and a sense of overall well-being from balancing your Qi. People often report an improved immune system and a greater ability to cope with daily stress.

Emotional Healing. The practice of Qigong can help heal your emotions and mind. It can help manage stress, anxiety, and depression, and increase self-awareness and empathy.

Spiritual Growth. Many people find Qigong to be deeply spiritual, connecting them to a greater sense of purpose. It can enhance one's connection to nature, the universe, and their inner self.

Pain Reduction. Qigong can reduce joint and muscle pain by improving mobility and reducing inflammation. Exercise like this is often recommended to people with chronic pain conditions.

Improved Circulation. Qigong helps to improve blood flow and stimulate lymphatic flow. This is important for getting rid of toxins and improving your health.

Qigong can indeed have these benefits, but everyone's experience will be different. As you practice, the benefits will accumulate over time, so practice regularly and with patience. Be sure you consult a doctor before beginning a new exercise routine if you have specific health issues. This section will give you an introduction to Qigong's history, principles, and holistic benefits. If you're looking for physical healing, emotional balance, or spiritual growth, Qigong can help.

Part 2

Step into the graceful world of Qigong, where each movement flows like a gentle stream, carrying away stress and infusing the body with vibrant energy. This is the art of transforming stillness into motion, merging breath with movement, and opening the door to a world of profound relaxation and energy development. In this section, we'll explore simple, yet powerful Qigong movements designed to enhance your energy flow and melt away stress, making the ancient wisdom of Qigong accessible to all, regardless of age or fitness level.

SIMPLE QIGONG MOVEMENTS

The Foundation: Understanding Qigong Posture and Breath

Qigong posture and breath work together to promote energy flow and well-being through physical alignment and mindful breathing

Posture - Keeping a correct posture is crucial to Qigong. A typical Qigong stance involves standing with feet shoulder-width apart, knees bent slightly (not extending beyond the toes), pelvis tucked slightly to straighten the lower back, and spine elongated. The shoulders should be relaxed, the chest open but not puffed out, and the arms should hang naturally. This Qigong Stance known also as "Zhan Zhuang" (standing like a post), connects you to the earth's energy and helps you ground yourself. Practicing this stance will improve your concentration, balance, increase stamina, and promote qi flow.

Breath. Qigong is about slow, deep, and mindful breathing, usually through the nose, focusing on the dentin about 2 inches below the navel. The navel, or belly button, is in the middle of your stomach area, between the bottom of your ribs and the top of your hips. It's the area where the umbilical cord was attached when you were in the womb. During inhalation and exhalation, the abdomen should expand and contract naturally. Also known as diaphragmatic breathing, it's great for calming the mind, reducing stress, and enhancing qi circulation.

Getting the posture and breath right is essential to harmonizing your body, mind, and spirit, promoting

91

health, and enhancing energy flow. These elements of Qigong form the basis of all Qigong exercises.

Conscious Breathing - Known as mindful breathing, it's about paying attention to your breath. Pay attention to how the breath moves through the body, noticing the rises and falls of the chest or belly, and feeling the air move through the nose or mouth. By being present with every breath, you'll calm your mind, reduce stress, and improve mental clarity. As you breathe, you're conscious of the patterns, depth, and speed. The breathing can involve deep belly breathing or controlled breaths, where you count or control the duration of each inhale and exhale. It's a great way to improve your awareness, reduce negative emotions, and feel good.

Beginning with the Basics - Qigong Warm-Up Exercises

Shaking the Body - It's often referred to as "Vibrational Qigong," where you shake and vibrate your whole body to release tension, improve circulation, and enhance your qi flow. It involves standing with

92

your feet shoulder-width apart, bending your knees slightly, and bouncing from your knees, allowing natural vibrations to travel up your body. Let your arms, shoulders, head, and the rest of your body shake naturally. The practice helps to relax muscles and joints, and can stimulate the body's energy pathways, promoting health and balance. This is typically done for a few minutes as a warm-up before other Qigong exercises or as a standalone exercise. Aside from it being believed to release stagnant energy, reduce stress, and promote emotional and physical release, it's also thought to help with fatigue and depression.

Arm Swings and Circles - To prepare your body and mind for practice, arm swings and circles enhance circulation and stimulate the flow of energy. This is how you typically do these exercises

Arm Swings - You want your feet to be shoulder width apart and your knees to be slightly bent. Arms and shoulders should be relaxed. Swing both arms forward and backwards gently without forcing the movement, allowing them to rise and fall naturally. Movement should come from the shoulders, not the arms. As your body warms up, you can gradually increase your range of motion. It releases tension in your shoulders and chest and stimulates blood and energy flow.

Arm Circles - From the same starting position, extend your arms out to the sides at shoulder height. Using your arms, make small circles, gradually getting bigger as your shoulders relax and warm up. Perform the circles in both a forward and a backward direction. You'll open your shoulders, improve your upper body circulation, and boost the flow of energy through your arms. It's great for loosening the upper body, promoting relaxation.

Here is a couple of Everyday Qigong Movements

Lifting the Sky - This Qigong exercise stretches and opens the body, promoting Qi (energy) flow from head to toe, and revitalizing the whole body.

Stand with your feet shoulder-width apart and your knees slightly bent.

Let your body relax, especially your arms and shoulders.

Place your hands in front of your lower abdomen, palms facing up, fingers slightly curled and pointing at each other as if you are holding a balloon.

As you breathe in, raise your hands above your head. As you reach your face, roll your hands over and push your palms up to the sky, gently stretching your body.

When your hands are overhead, open your arms to the side and gently lower them down.

Exhale as Pushing the Waves - Mimicking the ebb and flow of ocean waves, this movement helps balance emotions and strengthens the lower body while calming the mind. "Pushing the Waves" Qigong exercise:

Stand with your feet shoulder-width apart, one leg in front of the other. Knees slightly bent.

Keep your spine straight and relax your body.

As if pressing against a large ball, extend your arms in front of your chest, palms facing down and slightly forward.

As you inhale, shift your weight to your back leg and bring your arms close to your body, bending your elbows slightly and keeping your palms facing down.

As you exhale, shift your weight forward to your front leg, and gently push your palms forward and down, as if pushing waves away.

continue this back-and-forth motion in a soft fluid manner for a minute or two.

Keep your posture relaxed and focus on the smooth transition of weight between your legs, emulating the ebb and flow of waves.

Making movement a part of your daily life

Creating a Qigong routine that you can incorporate into daily living can help improve your overall well-being, energy levels, and mental clarity. A consistent practice of Qigong will nurture your mind and body.

You can follow this simple, adaptable routine

Get up in the morning and get going (5-10 minutes)

Gentle Stretching - Get your body awake with some gentle stretching. To loosen up, reach your arms overhead, stretch side to side, and gentle twist your torso.

Shaking the Body - You can release tension by shaking your whole body for a minute.

Lifting the Sky - To stretch your body and boost energy, do this exercise 6-8 times.

During lunchtime or break time (5 minutes): Refresh and rebalance

Pushing the Waves - Practice for 2-3 minutes to calm the mind and smooth out any emotional or energy blockages.

10-15 minutes in the evening: Unwind and reflect

Walking Qigong - Try to take a gentle walk outside. Breathe mindfully with every step.

Standing Meditation - With hands on your lower abdomen, stand quietly with your feet shoulder-width apart. Breathe deeply, letting stress go and relaxing.

Balancing the Qi - To end, imagine holding a ball of energy between your hands and moving it between your fingers to harmonize and balance your qi.

5 minutes before bed: Calm down and get ready for sleep

Child's Pose, also known as Balasana, is a gentle resting pose commonly used in yoga. It involves kneeling on the floor with your toes together and knees hip-width apart, then sitting back on your heels. From this position, you extend your arms forward on the floor and lower your forehead to the ground, fully stretching your back or Seated Forward Bend (A Seated Forward Bend is again a yoga pose where you sit with your legs extended in front of you and bend forward at the waist, reaching for your feet with your hands) - Choose a gentle, restorative pose to signal to your body it's time to wind down.

Breathing Exercise - Calm the nervous system and prepare for sleep by practicing deep abdominal breathing.

Don't forget to stay consistent. Qigong even for a few minutes can be helpful. Make it work for your schedule and practice at the same time every day to establish a rhythm. The purpose of this chapter was to introduce you to Qigong movements, so you can experience the power of aligning breath, body, and mind. There's more to these practices than just exercises; they are meditations in motion, portals to inner peace, and channels for the flow of life. Please take advantage of these gentle movements and let them guide you to strength, peace, and harmony. Welcome to the peaceful and energizing world of Qigong.

Part 3

No matter where you are or how little time you have, you'll always have a toolkit of tranquility at your fingertips. The essence of on-the-go Qigong is small, powerful practices that can be weaved seamlessly into your day, making even the most mundane moments a source of harmony and rejuvenation. In the middle of a busy day, waiting in line, or taking a break, these Qigong exercises are a great way to enjoy a moment of peace.

THREE ON-THE-GO EXERCISES FOR QIGONG

1. Shaking the Tree - A quick and energizing exercise that releases stress, loosens the joints and stimulates energy flow, perfect for reinvigorating the body after long periods of sitting or standing.

When to use it - Whenever you need to let go of physical and emotional tension, refuel yourself during a slump, or reset your nervous system after a stressful event. You can do this exercise anywhere you have a few feet of space and it's an effective way to release tension.

How to do it -

Stand with your feet shoulder-width apart and knees slightly bent.

100

Allow your arms to hang loosely by your sides.

You can start by gently bouncing off your knees, letting your arms shake naturally.

Increase the intensity slowly, shaking your whole body.

The whole time you're exercising, breathe deeply but naturally.

Let your shaking slow down after a minute or two.

Stand still for a moment, taking deep breaths, and notice the sensations in your body.

Benefits - A greater sense of well-being and relaxation, as well as reduced physical and emotional tension. Besides that, it can reset your nervous system, giving you a feeling of calm and grounding.

2. Pressing Heaven and Earth - Describing a powerful yet simple stretch that balances internal energies, stretches the body, and clears the mind, ideal for a refreshing break during a busy day.

When to use it - If you need to ease tension in your shoulders and spine, energize your body, improve your mental clarity, or transition between different activities, it's perfect. Perform this exercise in a quiet, spacious area, ideally where you won't be interrupted, such as a peaceful room at home or a calm outdoor environment, like a garden.

Practicing in the morning is a great time for energizing the body, while evening can help to unwind and relax.

How to do it -

Stand with your feet shoulder-width apart, knees slightly bent.

Start with your palms together in front of your chest in a prayer position.

Breathe deeply, then exhale while stretching both arms full out. One toward the earth and one upwards toward the sky. Keeping your palms facing away from you, push against two opposite forces.

Take a moment to feel the stretch on both sides of your body.

Breathe in as you bring your hands back to prayer position.

Then repeat the movement, but this time extend your opposite hand upwards and the other downward. Make sure that the motion is fluid and controlled

Alternate sides for several cycles, synchronizing your movements with your breath.

Benefits -

This helps with balance, coordination, blood flow, spinal flexibility, and shoulder and back tension. It also helps grounding and centering you, so you feel calm and balanced.

3. Five-Finger Qigong - It involves gentle finger movements and pressure points that relieve stress and improve concentration, even in crowded places. When to use it - When you feel mentally or physically tired, need to clear your mind, seek to balance your emotions, or during short breaks to revitalize and maintain focus throughout the day. It's discreet and quick, so you can do it anywhere, providing you with a moment of mindfulness at home or work.

How to do it -

Starting Position - Stand comfortably

Breathing and Focusing - Take a few deep breaths through your nose and out of your mouth to center yourself. Feel free to close your eyes if it's safe and if you want to. If you're in a crowd, you may not want anyone knowing.

Thumb Activation (Lung Meridian) - Spend about 30 seconds massaging the thumb pad. Then switch and do it on the other thumb. It's supposed to help with breathing problems and emotional distress.

Index Finger Activation (Large Intestine Meridian) - Then move on to your index finger, pressing and massaging its base for about 30 seconds. It's supposed to be good for digestion and backaches. The base of the index finger is the area where the finger meets the palm.

Middle Finger Activation (Pericardium Meridian) - This is supposed to make your heart healthy and emotional balance. Again, spend about 30 seconds doing this for each hand at the base.

Ring Finger Activation (Triple Burner Meridian) - Each hand, massage your ring finger base for about 30 seconds. This is associated with temperature and metabolic balance.

Little Finger Activation (Heart and Small Intestine Meridian) - Lastly, press and massage the base of your little finger for heart health and calm. Again, spend about 30 seconds on the little finger on each hand.

Closing - Shake your hands gently after you finish the finger exercises. Taking a few more deep breaths will help you relax and feel the energy flow through your body.

Benefits - Improved energy flow, stress reduction, enhanced focus and clarity, emotional balance, better physical health, and increased finger flexibility and strength. It's discreet so you can do it anywhere. On-the-go Qigong exercises help you balance daily stress with the peaceful flow of energy. Integrating these practices into your routine can give you strength and tranquility. Transform even the busiest days into opportunities for balance and wellness with this chapter. Explore the simplicity and power of Qigong and see how small changes can transform your mind and body.

CHAPTER 6

Part 1

EFT TAPPING: A TOOL FOR EMOTIONAL FREEDOM

How would you feel if you had a tool at your fingertips that could unlock emotional freedom and provide instant relief from life's stresses? The truth is, this is not the stuff of fantasy, but the reality of Emotional Freedom Techniques (EFT) Tapping. EFT Tapping is a revolutionary practice that combines ancient Chinese acupressure with modern psychology for powerful, transformative results that are unlike anything else out there. It is an easy, non-invasive, and very effective way to boost well-being by tapping into specific energy points on the body.

Understanding EFT Tapping

You can release emotional blockages by tapping on specific meridian points on your body and repeating affirmations or acknowledgment phrases.

The intention behind this process is to reduce stress, eliminate emotional distress, and promote healing at the same time. It involves tapping on certain points that are located on the head, face, and upper body, which correspond to the energy meridians used in the practice of acupuncture. There is an increasing use of EFT to help people with a variety of issues, such as anxiety, phobias, pain, and stress management. It offers a self-help approach to the regulation of emotions and relief of physical symptoms.

How EFT Tapping Works

Tapping combines cognitive therapy, exposure therapy, and acupressure. While tapping, repeat affirmations that acknowledge the issue and affirm self-acceptance. It works by reducing emotional stress and physical discomfort by altering the body's energy system. The EFT Tapping technique can help you cope better with negative emotions over time with repeated practice.

The Benefits of EFT Tapping

EFT tapping has gained wide popularity for its ability to provide significant relief and improvement across a range of mental and physical problems. Using a combination of traditional Eastern medicine principles and modern psychological therapies, the synergy offers a significantly unique approach to healing.

Reduced stress and anxiety - You can use EFT tapping to calm your nervous system, reduce cortisol, and get rid of anxiety symptoms. This makes it good for relaxing quickly and managing stress long-term.

Pain Management - Stress can cause a lot of physical pain. A lot of physical symptoms go away when you use EFT to address the psychological components of pain. It's beneficial for chronic pain conditions since it addresses both the physical sensation of pain and the emotional response to it.

Emotional Healing - Without feeling overwhelmed, EFT tapping lets you explore and heal emotional trauma. It is possible to lead healthier and more ful-filling lives by systematically addressing unre-solved emotional issues, thereby turning your life into one that is happier and less stressful.

Improvement in Mental Health - You can use EFT to treat depression, anxiety disorders, and phobias. As EFT encourages negative thought patterns to be altered, as well as reduced emotional distress, it can contribute to improving mental health and quality of life.

Boosted self-esteem - EFT can help uncover and ad-dress the root causes of low self-esteem, like past trauma or negative beliefs. Individuals can develop a more positive self-image and greater self-ac-ceptance by tackling these issues.

Reduction in cravings and addictions - The use of EFT helps reduce cravings and addictive behavior by addressing the emotional triggers. As a result, it's useful for promoting healthy lifestyles and manag-ing addictions.

110

Better Sleep - EFT tapping improves sleep by reducing stress and emotional distress, which are
common causes of insomnia. As a result of releasing these emotional blockages using tapping, individuals can enjoy a greater degree of relaxation and
find it easier to fall asleep and remain asleep
throughout the night.

Feeling energized - It's easy to feel tired and drained
when you've got emotional blockages. EFT can release these blockages, potentially increasing energy
and vitality. It has been reported that as the emotional health of an individual improves, they experience a sense of energy and vitality.

EFT tapping addresses issues both emotionally and
physically. It may vary from person to person, but
many find it an effective and empowering tool. Understanding EFT Tapping opens the door to a new
level of self-care. Using the techniques in this chapter, you'll be guided on your path to healing, bal-

ance, and emotional freedom. Discover the profound potential of EFT Tapping, a journey that puts you closer to peace and serenity.

Part 2

Imagine having a key to unlock the chains of stress and trauma, a method so straightforward yet profoundly impactful that it can be performed anytime, anywhere. This key is the EFT Tapping Routine, a series of steps designed to guide you through the process of emotional release and healing. Whether you're feeling the weight of daily stress or the deeper scars of past traumas, EFT Tapping provides a structured pathway to freedom, offering clarity, peace, and emotional balance. Let's walk through this routine together, step by step, as you learn to harness the power of tapping for a lighter, more blissful existence.

EFT TAPPING ROUTINE

The best way to prepare for your EFT session is to set an intention. Be clear about your goal and focus on one issue at a time for best results. Create a comfortable and private environment where you can relax and engage fully with the tapping process. Choose the morning to begin your day positively or evening to unwind. Decide which emotional issue or event you want to address, and how to articulate it clearly. From the top of the head to under the arm, locate and tap the key meridian points on the body. By repeating a concise phrase during tapping rounds, you can reinforce the process of releasing and resolving issues.

It's important to drink water after tapping because it is believed to help flush out toxins and waste products released from the cells. Hydration can enhance the effectiveness of a tapping session by supporting the body's natural healing processes. You are now one tap away from a calmer, more balanced you.

113

How to EFT tap

Identify the Issue - Decide what problem or emotion you want to focus on and rate it from 0-10.

Set up statement - Create a phrase acknowledging the issue and accepting yourself despite it, like "Even though I have this [issue], I deeply and completely accept myself."

Tapping - While repeating your phrase about your issue, gently tap each of the following meridian points for approximately a minute in this order

Karate Chop (Bottom side of the hand)

Eyebrow (Beginning of the eyebrow just above the nose)

Side of the Eye (Bone bordering the outside corner of the eye)

Under the Eye (Bone under the eye)

Under the Nose (Between the bottom of the nose and the top of the upper lip)

Chin (Crease below the lip and above the chin)

Beginning of the Collarbone (Where the sternum, collarbone, and the first rib meet)

Under the Arm (About four inches below the arm-pit)

Top of the Head (Centre of the top of the head)

Check the intensity again - Rate the intensity of your issue again after a few rounds. You can just repeat the tapping process if necessary, adjusting your phrases to reflect your current state or any new feelings.

Your meridian points and their meaning

Karate Chop (Small intestine Meridian. Bottom side of the Hand) - Used for the setup statement in EFT, often associated with clarity and decision-making.

Eyebrow (Bladder Meridian) - This is believed to affect the bladder meridian, which is associated with peace, emotional balance, and letting go.

Side of the Eye (Gallbladder Meridian) - Associated with the gallbladder meridian, this point helps re-lieve indecision and resistance.

Under the Eye (Stomach Meridian) - Located under the eye, this meridian represents the stomach. Tap-ping here is supposed to relieve stress and anxiety.

Under the Nose (Governing Vessel) - It's associated with self-acceptance and coping with negative emotions.

Chin (Central Vessel) - This meridian corresponds to the central meridian, so tapping here promotes clarity and peace.

Beginning of the Collarbone (Kidney Meridian) - Chinese medicine associates this point with the kidney meridian, which is related to fear and shock. Tapping here can help ease deep-seated fears and boost courage.

Under the Arm (Spleen Meridian) - This point is about a hand's width under the armpit, and it affects the spleen. It's good for lifting your mood, clearing worry, and dealing with resistance.

Top of the Head (Crown) - Spiritual connection and emotional calm are associated with this point, which affects the body's highest meridian.

As with any effective method of healing, EFT tapping is very efficient and can easily be integrated into everyday life to help address both emotional and physical issues. If you practice consistently, it's a great way to improve your mental health and physical comfort.

Part 3

In the rhythm of modern life, where each day whirls by filled with tasks, commitments, and unexpected challenges, finding a moment for emotional care might seem like a distant dream. Yet, what if relief and balance could be just a few taps away, no matter where you are or how limited your time might be? This is the power of on-the-go EFT Tapping exercises: quick, effective techniques designed to fit into any schedule, providing a fast track to emotional freedom and well-being, even amidst the busiest days.

THREE ON-THE-GO EXERCISES FOR TAPPING

1. The Quick Stress-Release Tap

When to use it - The perfect solution for moments when you feel stressed or anxious, like before a meeting or on the run during a full day of work.

How to do It - Use key tapping points to simplify the routine - karate chop, top of the head, eyebrow, and under the eye, combined with deep, calming breaths and a focus phrase like "Letting go of stress". This is typically performed for approximately 45 seconds per area. In most cases, this is enough to address immediate stress feelings. You can repeat the process if needed.

Benefits - It's great for reducing stress, clearing your head, and restoring your calm.

2. The Energy-Boost Tap

When to use it - This is perfect for battling midday fatigue or when you're feeling drained before an important task.

How to do It - Focus on tapping the top of the head, collarbone, and under the arm, while saying positive affirmations like "I welcome energy and focus."

Benefits - Increases alertness and combats lethargy, quickly stimulating the body and mind.

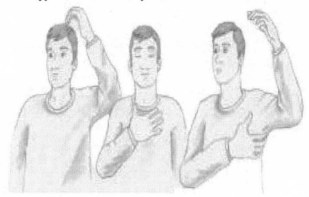

3. The Calm-Confidence Tap

When to use it - In situations where confidence and clarity are needed, like interviews, presentations, or difficult conversations.

How to do It - Tap on the karate chop, eyebrow, side of the eye, and under the nose while repeating affirmations like "I am calm and confident."

Benefits - Improves self-confidence and reduces anxiety, so you can approach challenges more calmly.

With these on-the-go EFT Tapping exercises, you can ensure emotional wellness doesn't fall by the wayside, no matter how busy your day is. It's all about maintaining balance, energy, and peace.

Exercise is a tool in your arsenal. Tap into your emotional freedom and self-care whenever you want with these simple and effective tapping techniques.

CHAPTER 7

Part 1

SOMATIC EXERCISES FOR DAILY LIFE

Imagine transforming every movement into a moment of discovery, where each step, stretch, and breath becomes a dialogue with your body. This is the art of Segmenting, a somatic exercise that invites you to break down everyday movements into smaller parts to enhance body awareness and deepen your connection to yourself. Whether you're brushing your teeth, walking to the store, or sitting at your desk, Segmenting teaches you to tune in to the differences of your physical experience, turning routine actions into opportunities for mindfulness and self-exploration.

Segmenting

Somatic segmenting is a therapeutic technique used to help individuals reconnect with their bodies and process emotions and sensations that may be stored

122

due to stress or trauma. It's grounded in somatic experiencing, a body-oriented approach to healing.

The process starts with bringing awareness to the
body and noticing physical sensations without judgment. This could involve scanning the body from
head to toe and recognizing areas of tension, discomfort, or numbness. The body is mentally divided
into segments (e.g., head, neck, shoulders, chest, abdomen, etc.). You focus on one segment at a time,
which can help manage overwhelming sensations
by dealing with them in smaller, more manageable
parts. Within each segment, you're encouraged to
explore sensations, emotions, and any associated
memories or thoughts. This exploration is done gently and gradually to avoid overwhelming the nervous system.

After focusing on individual segments, there's a
phase of integrating the experiences of each part
back into a sense of the whole body. This helps in
creating a new sense of coherence and wholeness.
Throughout the process, techniques for regulating

the nervous system are employed, such as deep breathing or grounding exercises, to ensure that the experience remains within a tolerable range of sensations.

Somatic segmenting helps individuals to gradually and safely experience and integrate previously intolerable bodily sensations and emotions, promoting healing and increased bodily awareness. It's typically used in the context of therapy with a trained professional.

So, what are the benefits of body awareness? By becoming more aware of bodily sensations associated with different emotions, you can recognize and address emotional states earlier, leading to better emotional regulation. Focusing on individual body segments helps break down overwhelming sensations into manageable parts, reducing overall stress and anxiety levels.

Understanding and feeling different parts of the body can help you distinguish between types of pain and develop strategies to manage it more effectively. Segmenting strengthens the connection between mind and body, leading to improved overall well-being and a deeper understanding of bodily signals. With increased body awareness, you can better understand your needs for rest, movement, or nutrition, promoting healthier lifestyle choices. For those dealing with trauma, segmenting allows for a gradual and safe exploration of trauma-related sensations and emotions, facilitating the healing process. Overall, increased body awareness through segmenting can lead to more mindful living, enhanced well-being, and a deeper sense of inner peace.

Applying segmenting to daily activities involves breaking down your experiences and tasks into smaller, more manageable parts, focusing on one segment at a time. This approach can enhance mind-fulness and reduce overwhelm. Here's how you can integrate it into your routine:

Morning Routine - Segment your morning into parts (waking up, showering, eating breakfast). Focus fully on each part as you do it, noticing the sensa-tions and experiences associated with each segment. For instance, feel the water during your shower, taste each bite of your breakfast.

Work or School Tasks - Break down your tasks into smaller segments. Focus on one small task at a time, fully engaging with it before moving to the next. This can help reduce feelings of overwhelm and in-crease productivity and focus.

Physical Exercise - During exercise, pay attention to different body parts as you move. For example, if you're walking or running, focus on your legs for a while, then your arms, and then your breathing. This helps in developing body awareness and can en-hance the benefits of exercise.

126

Eating - Segment your eating experience into smaller parts: looking at your food, smelling it, then slowly tasting each bite and experiencing its textures. This practice, often called mindful eating, can enhance the enjoyment of food and help with digestion.

Communicating - In conversations, break down the experience into listening and speaking. Focus fully on listening when the other person is talking, then on expressing yourself clearly when it's your turn. This can lead to more meaningful and effective communication.

Rest and Relaxation - Segment your relaxation time into different activities, such as reading, listening to music, or meditating. Focus fully on each activity for a set amount of time to deepen the relaxation experience.

By applying segmenting to your daily activities, you can become more present, reduce anxiety, and improve your overall quality of life.

Overcoming challenges with segmenting involves starting small and gradually increasing your practice as you become more comfortable. Remember the reasons you're incorporating segmenting into your routine, such as reduced stress or improved focus, and keep these benefits in mind as motivation. If you're feeling overwhelmed, reassess the size of your segments to make them more manageable. Use visual aids like sticky notes or alarms to remind you to practice segmenting throughout the day. Be flexible and adapt your approach when things don't go as planned. If you encounter resistance, try to understand the underlying reasons and address them. Sharing your goals with others can provide support and accountability. Recognize and celebrate your successes, however small, to boost motivation. Regularly reflect on your experiences, adjusting your approach as necessary. Most importantly, be patient and compassionate with yourself as you integrate this new habit into your life.

Over time, with consistent practice and adjustment, segmenting can become a natural and beneficial part of your daily routine.

Emphasize the importance of listening to your body's signals and respecting its limits. This will ensure that segmenting remains a gentle and enriching practice.

By inviting you to slow down and observe the intricacies of your movements,

Segmenting opens the door to a more mindful and connected way of living. This chapter serves as your guide to weaving increased body awareness into the fabric of your daily life, transforming ordinary actions into rich, somatic experiences. Embrace the practice of Segmenting, and watch as the world slows down, allowing you to live in deeper harmony with your body's rhythm and wisdom.

Part 2

When we understand what stress does to our body and how it reacts to perceived threats, we naturally move on to enhancing our sensory vocabulary. The more we can describe bodily sensations, the more self-aware we become and the more we heal. In the same way, as we are learning to navigate the stress cycle through somatic practices, expanding our sensory vocabulary will allow us to articulate and therefore better understand the subtle differences of our bodily experiences, allowing the vision to become tangible so that vague feelings can be understood.

SENSORY VOCABULARY EXPANSION

Expansion of our sensory vocabulary is like turning up the volume of the body-mind dialogue. In other words, we need to describe our experiences with detail and specifics, whether it's the gentle tension of anticipation or the warm flush of joy. Enhancing our vocabulary not only deepens our relationship with our bodies, but also enhances our emotional state. Having a more colorful palette gives us more freedom to express ourselves.

Here, we'll discuss the benefits of developing a rich sensory vocabulary and how it can enhance mindfulness and embodiment. By precisely naming our sensations, we can better understand our emotional and physical states and engage with our somatic practices.

To support this expansion, you can do exercises to sharpen your ability to describe bodily sensations. These include mindfulness practices that emphasize the sensations that can be felt within a single movement or breath, as well as journaling exercises that encourage descriptive exploration of somatic experiences, and guided interactions designed to help people share and clarify their experiences with others.

Building a rich sensory vocabulary makes communication more vivid and engaging. The more options you have for creative thinking and innovation, the more creative you can be. Also, this practice improves observational skills by getting a better sense of what's around you, which enriches your everyday life, and your interactions with nature and art. Also, it supports empathy since you know how other people feel and think.

A rich sensory vocabulary is crucial for memory, as sensory-rich memories are more vivid and lasting. Mindfulness and well-being are promoted by encouraging present moment awareness, which reduces stress and improves mental health.

For writers and artists, such vocabulary is invaluable for creating immersive, emotionally resonant works.

Through the study of language, people are also able to learn more about other cultures, thus enhancing personal understanding of different cultures.

In education, a rich sensory vocabulary supports multisensory learning, improving comprehension and retention for learners with diverse needs. It helps us understand and regulate our emotions by connecting them to sensory experiences. Having a rich sensory vocabulary enhances your cognitive skills, creativity, and personal relationships. By applying precise language to somatic practices, you enhance their effectiveness and deepen your overall body-mind connection.

The key to building a sensory vocabulary is to engage with and reflect on your senses actively. Start by immersing yourself in various environments, like nature, urban settings, art galleries or culinary experiences. Focus on the details of what you see, hear, feel, taste, and smell during these experiences. By reading widely, especially poetry and works from different cultures, you can discover new ways to express your senses. Trying to capture your senses in words through writing regularly also helps. It could be through creative writing or just taking notes.

Listening to and engaging in conversations about sensory experiences can also expand your vocabulary. If you discuss your perception of the same piece of music, food, or art with others, you may gain new perspectives and words you hadn't considered before.

It's also good to do practical exercises, like blindfolded taste tests or texture explorations. These can be fun and will sharpen your senses and make you find the words to describe your experiences. Engaging with art, music, and nature with a sensory focus can inspire new words.

Finally, studying the language itself - looking up synonyms, looking up thesaurus words, and exploring words in other languages that describe sensory experiences, can improve your sensory vocabulary. It's a continuous process of exploration, reflection, and expression aimed at capturing the richness of the sensory world.

In exploring sensory vocabulary expansion, we discover that the way we describe our bodily sensations is more than just words - it's a reflection of how closely we feel connected to our bodies.

This book encourages you to embrace the subtleties of your somatic experiences, using language to deepen your awareness. It is through this practice that you will find that each of your sensations, each of your movements, will be a word in the ongoing story, enriching and enlarging your journey toward healing and wholeness.

Part 3

We're building on the sensory vocabulary expansion, but now it's time to apply it in our everyday lives. Our journey here focuses on incorporating somatic practices into daily routines, making living an embodied, conscious act.

Even amidst our busy lives, segmenting exercises during routine activities, like walking or sitting, will develop mindfulness and deepen our connection to our bodies.

THREE ON-THE-GO EXERCISE FOR SEGMENTING EXERCISES DURING ROUTINE ACTIVITIES

1. Walking with Awareness

When to use it - When you're walking, whether you're running errands, exercising, commuting, or just taking a break.

How to do it -

Start with Intention - Put a goal for your walk in your head. It could be as simple as being present during the walk or taking a stress break.

Focus on Your Breathing - Before you start walking, take a few deep breaths. As you inhale and exhale, take a moment to notice the sensation of the air moving into your lungs. This prepares you for mindful walking.

Pay Attention to Your Steps - When you start walking, focus on how your legs and feet feel. Take note of how your feet feel on the ground, how the weight shifts from one foot to the other, and how your steps flow.

Engage Your Senses - Be aware of what's around you, including the sights, sounds, smells, and textures. Feel the air on your skin, notice the colors you see, the sounds you hear, and the scents you smell. Feel these sensations like you're experiencing them for the first time.

Observe Your Surroundings - Be aware of your surroundings, whether it's a busy street, a quiet neighborhood, or a natural trail. Pay attention to the details without labelling or judging them. Simply notice and appreciate the world around you.

Acknowledge Distractions - Wandering minds happen. When you find your mind drifting to the past or the future, gently acknowledge it and put your focus back on walking.

Use Gentle Reminders - To maintain focus, you may be able to silently remind yourself with each step, "right, left, right" or synchronize your steps with your breath by thinking "in" and "out,".

Conclude with Gratitude - When you're done walking, slow down and appreciate the experience, your ability to walk, and the time you've taken for your-self.

Benefits - Helps lower stress and anxiety, boosts focus and mood, and improves physical health. Using it as a stress management tool deepens your connection with the environment and increases self-awareness.

An automatic activity like walking becomes a conscious practice of movement. A mindful stroll turns a routine activity into a meditation practice, enhancing your connection to the present moment and the subtleties of your body.

2. Mindful Sitting

When to use it - During breaks, before important events, and when you're stressed to keep things in perspective. When you're switching between activities to stay present, and at the beginning or end of your day to set a good tone. Anytime you sit, it's an opportunity to practice and improve your well-being.

138

How to do it -

Find a Quiet Space - Sit somewhere peaceful without distractions.

Choose a Seat - Place your feet flat on the ground or cross your legs. You can choose whichever feels more comfortable.

Adopt a Posture - Keep a comfortable upright posture with your hands on your lap.

Close Your Eyes or Soften Gaze - Visual distractions are reduced this way.

Focus on Breath - Listen to your natural breathing rhythm, noticing the sensations of air moving through you.

Notice Body Sensations - Be aware of your physical feelings without judging them. It means observing them with openness and compassion.

Acknowledge Thoughts and Emotions - Watch your thoughts and emotions come and go without engaging them.

Return to Breath - Refocus on your breathing when you're distracted.

Conclude with Gratitude - Thank yourself for practicing.

Benefits - Relieves stress, improves focus and emotion regulation, enhances mindfulness, and promotes well-being. During a busy day, it's a great way to clear your head.

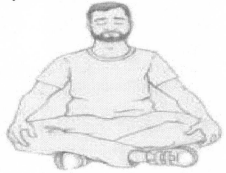

3. Typing with Awareness

When to use it - You can do it during work or study sessions to enhance focus, during creative writing to deepen engagement, and whenever you're typing to improve accuracy.

How to do it -

Begin with Intention - Put a goal on your typing task. It could be staying focused, typing mindfully, or connecting deeply with what you're writing.

140

Prepare Your Space - Keep your typing area organized to minimize distractions. Keep your space clear to keep your mind clear.

Notice Your Posture - Your back should be straight, your feet flat on the floor, and your hands gently resting on the keyboard. You'll be more alert and feel more relaxed when you have a good posture.

Breathe Mindfully - Taking a few deep breaths before you begin will help you focus. You'll be able to pay attention more mindfully when you do this.

Feel the Keys - Try paying attention to what it feels like when your fingers are pressing the keys. Notice the rhythm of your typing and the feel of each keystroke.

Observe Your Thoughts and Emotions - Think about how you're feeling as you type. Just acknowledge your feelings without judging them and go back to typing.

Take Regular Breaks - Pause now and then to stretch and breathe deeply. By doing this, you'll be able to keep your focus and avoid physical strain.

Conclude with Gratitude - Once you've finished typing, take a moment to appreciate the work you've done and the mindfulness you practiced.

Benefits - Practicing typing with awareness can help you type faster and more accurately, reduce physical strain, and improve your mental clarity. Your work feels more personal, leading to better productivity and creativity, while also helping you manage stress and stay focused.

It is exciting to realize that as we embrace these on-the-go segmenting exercises into our daily lives, we can see how somatic awareness is not limited to the boundaries of formal practice but rather is a way of being, accessible at anytime, anywhere. Upon realizing these truths, we are allowed to enter a new world, one where every step, every breath becomes an opportunity to be mindful and to grow. The purpose of these exercises is to gently invite you to inhabit your body more fully, to transform routine activities into a dance of awareness and presence, and to bring to life the principles of somatic therapy over the course of your regular life.

CHAPTER 8

Part 1

TECHNIQUES FOR DEEPENING THE MIND-BODY CONNECTION

A s we move beyond the foundational practices of somatic therapy, we explore the powerful effects of movement, dance, and expressive arts. The story takes us into a dynamic space where the body's language is not only heard but celebrated, allowing us to express emotion, heal, and deepen the connection between the mind and body.

Exploring Movement and Dance

Movement and dance are more than physical activities; they're expressions of our innermost thoughts, feelings, and experiences. When we move our bodies freely, without judgement or constraint, we tap into deep reservoirs of emotion and memory. There's an inseparable relationship between mind and body in movement and dance therapy. By moving and dancing, you can express yourself in ways

144

words can't capture, bridging the gap between traditional talk therapy and the subconscious mind.

Techniques and Practices

Experimenting with free movement - Letting your
body lead the way as you move unstructured to music or silence. In this practice, you listen to your
body's impulses and let go of your emotions.

Guided Imagery and Movement - With a combination of visualization and movement, this technique
creates a deeper connection with the emotional and
symbolic content of our inner world by influencing
the movement of our bodies in response to specific
prompts or images.

Performing rituals and group dances - Taking part
in ritualistic or ceremonial movement activities that
promote community, shared experience, and collective healing.

Integrating Expressive Movement into Daily Life
By incorporating expressive movement into daily
life, you'll improve your physical and mental health.

You don't need a dance studio or formal dance training to incorporate expressive movement and dance into your daily routine.

Start Your Day with Movement - Set a positive tone for the day by dancing or stretching to music you love.

Take Movement Breaks - Try taking short breaks throughout the day to stretch, dance, or do anything that feels good. It'll boost your energy and make you feel better.

Use Music as a Cue - Let your body move to the rhythm of music that resonates with your mood or how you want to feel. This helps you express and process emotions.

Incorporate Movement into Routine Activities - Whenever you're doing household chores or routine tasks, add expressive movements like reaching, bending, or dancing.

Practice Mindful Walking - During walks, vary your pace, notice how your body feels while you move, and maybe even add in some playful steps or stretches.

Spend time in nature - Make the most of the natural setting when you're outside. Try stretching towards the sun, balancing on a log, or swaying in the breeze.

End Your Day with Gentle Movement - To unwind before bed, do gentle, expressive movements like yoga or slow dancing.

When we explore movement and dance through the lens of therapeutic practices, we discover that they have the unique ability to promote the release of emotional tension. Movements, especially sponta-neous ones, can help release emotions frozen in the body, opening a powerful and gentle pathway to healing. Through movement and dance we are re-minded of the body's inherent wisdom and ability to heal. The purpose of this section of the book is to inspire you to embrace the expressive potential of your body, find freedom and grace in movement, and discover the transformative power of dance as a path to a deeper comprehension of yourself and a deeper connection to others. Let your body's rhythm lead you toward a more expressive and vibrant existence.

Part 2

Through movement and dance, we move naturally into breathwork for emotional depth and freedom of expression. Our breath has the power to access, illuminate, and release deep-seated emotions that reside within us. Using the breath as a key, it is like taking a journey inward, inside ourselves, revealing parts of us that are often hidden from our conscious awareness. This provides a pathway to healing that is both gentle and powerful at the same time.

BREATH WORK FOR EMOTIONAL DEPTH

Our physical and emotional worlds are deeply connected through breathwork. With advanced breathing techniques, we can explore the depths of our emotional landscape, releasing tension, trauma, and blockages held in our bodies. Breathing is our most constant companion, an ever-present tool for influencing our brain and body.

Through advanced breathwork techniques, we can lead ourselves through emotional breakthroughs and deep healing.

Advanced Breathwork Techniques Explored

Holotropic Breathwork - Developed around the 1970s by psychiatrists Stanislav Grof and Christina Grof, Holotropic Breathwork (HBW) is a therapeutic breathing method that achieves altered states of consciousness without the use of any substances whatsoever. This practice involves accelerated breathing patterns, which can alter consciousness, letting practitioners' access and work through emotional and psychological stuff that's hidden from day-to-day awareness. It combines accelerated breathing with evocative music and a supportive setting to unlock emotions and memories. The purpose of it is to support self-discovery, growth, and healing. It's based on the belief that individuals have an innate healing wisdom within them. The intense nature of this practice means it's best practiced with a certified instructor, especially if you have health issues.

The following is a simplified overview of how it typically done

Setting - The practice is done in a safe, supportive group setting, led by trained instructors. The participants pair up, one breathing, the other being the emotional support.

Preparation - Participants often start with some form of bodywork or group activities to relax. This could be something like stretching. Each person sets an intention for their session.

Breathing Technique - As the "breather" lies on a mat, he or she closes their eyes or wears an eye mask. Concentrate on deep, rapid breathing, which will help you build energy.

Music and Sound - During the session, an in-depth playlist of music is provided which ranges from meditative to highly energetic, all of which have

been carefully selected to evoke emotional responses and support the participants inner journey.
Experience and Expression - Throughout the session, participants may experience a lot of sensations
and visions. Movement, vocalizations, and emotional releases are encouraged as part of the process.
Integration - After the breathing phase, participants
draw or share stories to integrate their experiences.
Closure - It ends with a return to normal consciousness and a conversation about the experience, often
sharing insights or emotional breakthroughs.

Rebirthing Breathwork - Also known as Conscious
Energy Breathing, is a technique developed by
Leonard Orr. You can release emotional energy ac-
cumulated from birth trauma and early life experiences with this technique. Breathing is continuous
and connected without pauses between inhalations
and exhalations. People often feel emotional and
physical releases, gain more self-awareness, and
sometimes have mystical experiences. Based on the
belief that breath is a life force that heals our bodies

and minds, breathing techniques can lead to deep emotional and spiritual change.

Considering the intensity and potential for deep emotional experiences, Rebirthing Breathwork should be done by an experienced practitioner, especially if you're new to breathwork or have underlying health issues.

To give you a brief overview, here's how it's done Environment Setup - This practice usually takes place in a comfortable, private setting. The participants can lie down or sit comfortably to allow uninterrupted breathing.

Breathing Technique - It's all about conscious, connected breathing. The participants breathe in and out continuously, without pausing. It's mostly done through the nose, which promotes a higher energy intake and a meditative state.

Guidance - A practitioner guides the participant, offering verbal cues and support to help maintain breathing rhythms, navigate emotional releases, and stay focused.

Emotional Release - Using this technique, suppressed emotions and memories can surface, sometimes from early childhood or birth. The participants are encouraged to express these emotions.

Integration - Following the active breathing portion, there's a period of reflection and relaxation. In this way, the participant can integrate the knowledge and insights learned.

Sharing and Discussion - A practitioner may offer further guidance and sharing of experiences after the session, aiding in the integration process.

Transformational Breathwork - Developed by Dr. Judith Kravitz in the 1970s, this method combines yoga, meditation, and other healing practices. Through full, diaphragmatic breathing, affirmations, sound, and movement, it helps clear blockages and heal emotional wounds. It's a holistic healing technique that helps you feel better physically, emotionally, and spiritually. The goal is to help individuals access deeper levels of self-awareness and release suppressed traumas. It's great for bringing

about significant and, as the name implies, transformational changes. There are millions of people
practicing it throughout the world, and it's accessible to all ages and levels of physical fitness. Book a
session with a certified instructor If you're exploring
breathwork for the first time or have specific health
concerns.

Here's a concise overview

Breathing Pattern - In this practice, you take deep,
continuous breaths without pauses between inhalations and exhalations. Emphasis is on breathing
fully and freely, engaging the diaphragm, and using
all your lungs.

Posture and Setting - You can do it lying down, sitting, or even standing. Music and sometimes aroma-
therapy enhance the experience by creating a comfortable and supportive atmosphere.

Instructor Role - An instructor guides the participant through the session, offering feedback and
hands-on techniques to open parts of their breathing

pattern that are restricted. They will constantly monitor your comfort and safety.

Physical Release - Intense breathing techniques are designed to enhance the flow of oxygen and energy in the body, thereby reducing tension, alleviating chronic pain, and possibly improving any health conditions.

Emotional and Psychological Healing - The release of suppressed emotions and limiting beliefs can lead to significant shifts in mood, reduced stress, and a greater sense of happiness.

Spiritual Connection - Practitioners report a deeper sense of purpose and interconnectedness during sessions, as well as profound spiritual connection.

Integration Phase - Following active breathing, the body and mind are allowed to relax and take in the session's experiences.

Reflection and Sharing - During group settings, participants may share insights or breakthroughs about their experiences.

The best way to integrate advanced breathwork into your practice is to establish a solid foundation in basic techniques. Learning through workshops and courses is an excellent way to deepen your understanding of the subject. Practicing regularly is important to see the effects first-hand, which is invaluable when guiding others. Introduce advanced breathing techniques gradually, paying attention to how you or others react, since they can trigger strong emotional and physical reactions. Making sure everyone is safe and ensuring a supportive environment is always a priority. Integrating and reflecting after practice are crucial to processing profound insights and emotions. Getting feedback and sharing experiences with mentors can enrich your practice. Recognize that everyone's journey is different, so customize practices accordingly. Respect confidentiality, and boundaries, and always keep a nonjudgmental attitude. Breathwork practices from foundational to advanced enhance personal growth and the ability to help others.

The role of breath in emotional release is transform-ative.

As a bridge between mind and body, the breath al-lows us to access, process, and release stored emo-tions. When these emotions are suppressed, they may manifest in the form of tension, blockages, or pain in the body. Using conscious breathing tech-niques helps release these blockages, allowing emo-tions to surface.

By breathing deeply and intentionally, you can shift your body's state from stress and anxiety to relaxa-tion and openness. This shift is due to the activation of the parasympathetic nervous system, which pro-motes relaxation and healing. It's easier for the mind to let go of control in this state.

Breathwork helps release emotional baggage that's been held in your tissues by encouraging the flow of oxygen and energy through your body.

People who practice breathwork often experience cathartic releases, like crying, laughing, or singing.

The process helps rid the body of pent-up emotional stress, making you feel lighter, clearer, and happier. By practicing advanced breathwork, you learn that your breath can act as a bridge between your conscious and subconscious minds, between your physical sensations and your deepest emotions. Through it, we can uncover deep emotions and memories within us, providing insights that are both reflective and revealing.

By exploring breathwork for emotional depth, we embrace a powerful tool for healing and self-discovery. Using our breath to access and release deep-seated emotions invites profound changes in our relationship with ourselves. The practices in this segment will help you explore the depths of your emotional landscape with courage and curiosity, using the breath as your guide.

Part 3

Transitioning from the foundational practices of breathwork for emotional depth, we now venture into practical applications that can be effortlessly integrated into daily life. This section introduces three on-the-go exercises designed to synchronize breath with movement, encouraging emotional release and deepening the mind-body connection in accessible, tangible ways. These exercises exemplify how the principles of somatic therapy can be applied to everyday activities, turning ordinary moments into opportunities for healing and mindfulness.

THREE ON-THE-GO EXERCISES: BREATH SYNCHRONISATION WITH MOVEMENT FOR EMOTIONAL RELEASE

1. Mindful Walking with Breath

When to use it - It's perfect for walking anywhere, taking a short break outside, or even taking a quiet stroll in the garden.

How to do it - Choose a regular walking route, such as your commute to work or a lap around your backyard. Establish a breathing pattern that matches your steps (for example, inhale for four steps, hold for two, exhale for four steps, hold for two). Concentrate on the sensation of air moving in and out of your lungs, and how your feet feel against the ground. Use the exhale to release any tension or emotions that surface.

Benefits - You'll feel grounded, reduce stress, and harmonize the body's movements with the breath, promoting a sense of inner balance and emotional release.

2. Stretching with Focused Breathing

When to use it - Before your day starts, after exercise like walking or jogging, or during short breaks at work. It's also great for transitioning between tasks.

How to do it - Try a simple stretch like reaching for the sky or gently twisting your torso. During the motion, breathe in as you extend or twist, and exhale as you return to the starting position. Imagine tension melting away with every exhale as you focus on the sensations in your muscles and joints.

Benefits - It enhances flexibility and helps unpack emotions in tight spots in the body, facilitating relaxation and emotional clarity.

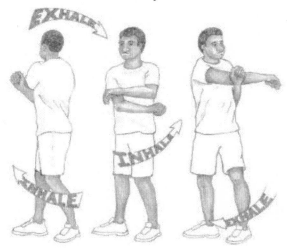

3. Synchronized Breathing with Household Chores
When to use it - As you do everyday tasks like washing dishes, vacuuming, or tidying.

How to do it - Choose a repetitive chore, like folding laundry or doing dishes. Set up a breathing rhythm that matches your actions (for instance, breathe in as you fold and exhale as you put something down). Become meditative by letting your attention rest on your physical sensations and your breath.

161

Benefits - Reduces stress, increases presence and calm, and helps reduce anxiety. As a result of combining focused breath and movement in this exercise, mundane tasks become moments of mindfulness that dissolve stress and emotional buildup, allowing us to regain our focus and energy.

It is evident from these on-the-go exercises, that the journey to emotional freedom and the development of a deeper mind-body connection does not require a significant departure from our everyday lives, but instead, a conscious engagement with them to make these changes possible. It is through synchronizing your breath with your movement that you can invite moments of mindfulness into your daily routine and leverage the therapeutic power of somatic practices to navigate life's challenges with greater ease and resilience. Make these exercises part of your self-care routine. Let your body be your guide to a more harmonious, emotionally balanced life.

CHAPTER 9

Part 1

CULTIVATING RESILIENCE AND WELL-BEING

The journey to holistic well-being involves cultivating resilience, which guides us through life's inevitable storms. As this chapter explores the heart of somatic practice, it gives you strategies to sustain and deepen your connection to your body, to boost your strength, endurance and well-being. Keep in mind: building a consistent and enriching somatic practice is both a journey and a destination; it's about connecting with our deepest parts and discovering ourselves on the way.

Building a Somatic Practice

A somatic journey invites us to be aware, compassionate, and curious about our bodies. It builds resilience in us and provides a stable foundation for navigating life's challenges with grace and agility. The first thing we do is set up a routine. Start by integrating somatic exercises into your day, at times that feel natural to you.

Consistency is key to developing a sustainable practice, whether it's a morning stretch, midday breathing break, or evening wind-down. Create a dedicated space. If possible, designate a specific area in your home as your somatic practice space. There's no need for it to be big or elaborate, just a corner of a room or a comfortable chair will do. Personalize your practice. You can customize your somatic exercises based on your preferences and needs. There's no right or wrong way to use different techniques and the most important thing is to find what feels most beneficial and enjoyable for you. Reflect on your experience after each session. Keep track of any sensations, emotions, or thoughts that arise. Through this reflection, you will gain a deeper understanding of yourself and enhance the connection between your body and yourself. Stay on top of somatic theories and practices. Learn how the body reacts to stress, trauma, and healing so you can understand and engage with it better. If you want to keep your practice lively and engaging, you should present new exercises or variations from time to time. This could include exploring different types of movement, integrating breath work, or trying somatic therapies like Qigong or dance which we talked about previously. Being part of a community of like-minded people provides encouragement, inspiration, and a sense of belonging. Join a somatic practice group, workshop, or class. When you share your experiences with others, you get a better understanding and are more committed. Sharing your journey can be affirming and inspiring,

The act of building a somatic practice shows self-love and commitment to your wellbeing. It's about honoring your body and about cultivating a resilient spirit that can embrace life with openness and strength. Don't underestimate the power of curiosity, compassion, and an unwavering belief in your potential for growth and transformation.

165

This is about helping you develop a practice that sustains you through life's ups and downs and enhances your life with joy, depth, and profound well-being.

Part 2

Having built a resilient, well-being-focused somatic practice, we're now going to weave these practices seamlessly into everyday life. Living a somatic lifestyle doesn't just involve isolated exercises or moments of mindfulness; it's about integrating these practices into every aspect of your life, letting them influence your interactions, decisions, and overall approach to living.

INTEGRATING SOMATIC PRACTICES INTO DAILY LIFE: MAKING SOMATICS A LIFESTYLE

Adapting somatic practices into a fully integrated lifestyle takes mindfulness and commitment. The idea is to engage with your body in a meaningful way, in every moment, nurturing a continuous dialogue between mind and body.

Make somatic exercises part of your daily routine, like stretching while your coffee brews or practicing mindful breathing on the way to work. The good news is that these practices can become as habitual as brushing your teeth. Practicing somatic awareness at meals. Make eating a sensory experience, from the texture and taste of your food to chewing and swallowing. It'll boost digestion and satisfaction. Instead of a typical coffee break, introduce movement or breathing breaks. Spend a few minutes stretching, doing qigong movements, or mindful walking to rejuvenate your mind and body. You should take care of your emotional and mental health through daily somatic practices just like you take care of your physical body. Writing down your feelings, checking in with your physical sensations, or setting breathwork intentions can help you release your emotions. During conversations, pay attention to how your body reacts.

How do you feel physically? Are you stressed or relaxed? You can change the dynamics of the conversation by changing your posture, breathing, or talking pace. Make your living and working space somatic-friendly. It might mean creating spaces that encourage movement, adding elements that engage the senses, like plants or art, or designing your seating to support good posture.

Somatics Rituals

Morning and Evening Routines - Ritualize your day to start and end. For example, in the morning you might include a yoga practice or dynamic stretching to energize your body, whereas in the evening, you might engage in calming practices such as deep breathing or gentle qigong to help you relax.

Responsive Somatics - Learn how to respond to different emotions with somatic practices. Think of tension-release exercises for stress, grounding techniques for anxiety, and energizing movements for lethargy.

When you integrate somatic practices into everyday life, you turn body awareness from a practice into a lifestyle.

With this holistic approach, you're not only going to feel better physically and emotionally but also build stronger relationships, and interactions with the world will be clearer and more focused. Make these principles a part of your lifestyle and see how they lead to a more balanced, joyful, and connected life.

Part 3

Our next step is to explore the power of community in deepening somatic practices. The benefits of group exercises, like Qigong and synchronized breathing, are endless, from promoting connection to enhancing well-being. As well as strengthening individual practices, these community exercises create shared experiences that connect participants emotionally and energetically.

THREE ON-THE-GO EXERCISES: GROUP QIGONG OR SYNCHRONISED BREATHING FOR COMMUNITY CONNECTION

1. Circle Qigong

When to use it - In a group setting, like before yoga or a club meeting. To make sure no stress is put on the group, the timing should complement the club's purpose.

How to do it - Stand shoulder to shoulder in a circle. Start by doing a simple Qigong warm-up, synchronizing your breath with gentle arm raises. (The art of Qigong is discussed in Chapter 5). Inhale when the arms are raised, exhale when they're lowered.

Play "Passing the Ball," where you pass and receive an energy ball around the circle. Three to five rounds work best for deeper engagement, allowing the energy to build and participants to refine their skills. You can adjust the number of rounds based on the number of participants, the available time, and the size of the group.

170

Benefits - It builds a sense of unity and shared purpose between participants, deepening their connection through energy flow.

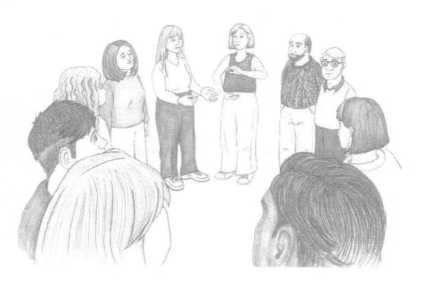

2. Harmonized Breath Walk

When to use it - Organize a group walk in nature or a quiet park. Places with lots of open space, like beaches or fields.

How to do it - Synchronize your breathing and walking pace. You can do this by breathing in for three steps and breathing out for three steps. Now and again, you can stop to spend a moment holding hands, breathing deeply, and sharing stillness. One

171

to three minutes is usually enough. Have fun with your senses. Get lost in the moment.

Benefits - The result is a deeper connection with nature and each other, which is calming and creates a feeling of peace and alignment for everyone.

3. Ripple Breath Exercise

When to use it - In yoga studios or meeting rooms which are quiet indoor spaces where participants can sit or stand near to enhance collective energy. Group breathing exercises can also be done in a calming outdoor environment such as a park or garden, where nature is part of the practice.

How to do it - Sit or stand in a circle and focus on the breath. One person starts by taking a deep breath and on the exhale, the next person begins their inhale. In this way, the breathing ripples around the circle. Again, depending on time and how many people are in a group, 3-5 times around the circle usually works.

Benefits - As everyone feels intimately connected to everyone else's breath, they develop emotional empathy and teamwork, which leads to collective relaxation.

Incorporating these group exercises into regular meetups or special events can significantly enhance the community's overall well-being. It's a powerful reminder of how interconnected we are and how strong we are when we all pull together to heal. Whether they're in a yoga studio, a community center, or a quiet spot in a park, these practices create a supportive network that lasts beyond the exercises. Why does community practice matter? Getting involved in somatic practices with others brings a lot of energy and perspective, which can lead to deeper emotional and physical insights. They eliminate feelings of isolation by creating connections and amplifying the healing intentions of everyone, creating a powerful, shared wellness journey. Through these community-centered exercises in Qigong and synchronized breathing, you can build a supportive, empathetic community that bonds over the rhythm of breath and movement.

By embracing these practices, you will be able to experience the impact of collective somatic work, enriching your journey towards living a deeply connected strong life.

CHAPTER 10

Part 1

TRANSFORMING LIFE THROUGH SOMATIC AWARENESS

We are in the midst of a transformational journey for somatic practices, and the power of personal stories that comes with them is a testimony to the underlying power that emerges when we deepen our connection to our bodies as a way of healing and growing. The following case studies of real-life transformations serve not only as proof of the effectiveness of somatic therapy but also as inspiration to those who are looking for healing, a deeper understanding of themselves, and a better understanding of the world around them.

Case Studies

As you read through the stories in this section, it becomes clear that somatic practices can be an encouragement for significant changes in a person's life, bringing an emotional connection to the principles and exercises discussed throughout this book.

Maria: Healing from Chronic Anxiety

Maria, a 34-year-old graphic designer, had battled with anxiety for most of her adult life. Her condition was not well treated by traditional therapies, and it interfered with her work and relationships. It was through a combination of mindful movement exercises and guided breathing exercises that Maria learned to manage her symptoms by tuning into her body's signals and using breath as a tool to calm her mind in moments of high anxiety. With time, she was able to deepen her practice, which led to a significant decrease in her levels of anxiety and an improvement in the quality of her life.

James: Overcoming Physical and Emotional Trauma

A serious car accident left James, a 45-year-old teacher with persistent back pain and emotional trauma, including PTSD. It seemed to him that he was disconnected from his body, which caused him pain and frustration. He was able to re-establish trust in his body through somatic experiencing therapy, which included pendulation and titration techniques. Taking this approach helped him process and integrate his traumatic experiences, resulting in both physical and emotional improvements.

Anita: Finding Balance with Qigong

The physical demands of ageing and the emotional drain of having three kids weighed heavily on Anita, a 66-year-old retired nurse. She discovered Qigong in a community class and liked its gentle, rhythmic movements and focus on breath and energy flow. The reason she loved practicing Qigong was that it gave her relief from physical pain and a sense of calm that had never been felt before. Having a supportive and engaging environment in a community class really helped her get the most out of Qigong.

Elena: Reclaiming Life After Depression

Elena, a 29-year-old social worker, had suffered from severe depression for years. Because of her condition, she had a hard time maintaining relationships and working efficiently. In an attempt to achieve some improvement, Elena turned to somatic therapy as a last resort when traditional therapy and medication failed to provide any results. With regular expression dance therapy and breath work, Elena's mood and outlook started changing. By expressing herself physically, she could release pent-up emotions, while her breathing rhythmically helped her relax. As she continued to practice these techniques, her depressive symptoms began to subside, and she began to regain hope and joy that had been missing for years.

Tom: Enhancing Performance and Reducing Stress

In this case, Tom, a 50-year-old executive, faced high levels of stress on a daily basis, which negatively affected his health and performance at the work. Despite a successful career, Tom was constantly physically and emotionally exhausted and overwhelmed. Then a coworker introduced him to somatic exercises for stress management. To manage his stress, Tom used EFT on-the-go tapping and targeted mindfulness exercises throughout the day. In addition to lowering his heart rate and reducing muscle tension, these practices helped him make better decisions and think clearly. This resulted in Tom experiencing a significant improvement in the level of his professional performance and personal satisfaction, allowing him to thrive at any time and under any circumstances.

These stories illuminate the journey from struggle to healing and balance, highlighting the power of somatic awareness and consistent practice. Their insights highlight the importance of a personalized approach: Recognizing that everyone's healing path is different. Incorporating somatic practice into everyday life will show how it can aid in managing and alleviating both physical and emotional distress. Body-focused therapy like mindfulness movement, guided breath work, and somatic experiencing can be transformative, as Maria and James show us. The practices help people reconnect with their bodies, manage anxiety and trauma symptoms, and improve both their mental and physical health. It shows how important holistic approaches are when dealing with health issues. Supportive groups can also play a big role in sustaining and enhancing personal growth and well-being, as Anita showed. As seen in Elena's journey, engaging the body in creative and expressive ways can tap into feelings that traditional therapies might not reach. In Tom's case, somatic practices can be adapted to the corporate world, providing stress management tools for professionals.

180

Reflecting on these narratives, we recognize that transforming ourselves through somatic awareness doesn't only mean that we will be able to overcome ailments, but also that we will embrace a holistic way of living that will improve all aspects of our lives. There is a potential for change within each one of us, reinforced through the stories, which teach us to become in tune with our bodies and find our own path to healing. As we read in the case studies, there are all kinds of applications for somatic practices, from dealing with mental health issues to dealing with work stress. It is through these narratives that we can gain not just a glimpse into individual journeys of healing and growth, but also to serve as a guide to encourage readers to explore and fuse these practices into their own lives, enhancing strength, well-being, and a deeper connection to their bodies.

Part 2

After hearing inspiring stories of transformation and healing through real-life case studies, let's talk about how to apply these somatic practices in real life. Developing a sustained lifestyle of somatic awareness invites a shift in habits and how we live and interact with the world.

INTEGRATING SOMATIC PRACTICES INTO DAILY LIFE

When you adopt somatic practices as a lifestyle, you turn routine actions into opportunities for self-awareness and healing. We're trying to make a life that not only accommodates but is enriched by somatic therapy principles. Make somatic practices part of your daily routine. It could be as simple as stretching while the coffee brews or practicing mindful breathing in the shower. These practices should be as much a part of your day as eating and sleeping. Prepare yourself for daily stress by learning specific somatic responses. For instance, if you feel overwhelmed at work, have a go-to breathing technique or a brief series of stretches that help center and calm you. It not only mitigates stress, but also enhances your ability to deal with challenges. Take short somatic breaks throughout the day. It could be three minutes of deep breathing, a meditation session, or even some light Qigong. When you're facing a busy, challenging day, it's essential to take breaks to maintain your energy and focus.

Interacting socially with somatic awareness

Improve your listening skills by using somatic awareness. Pay attention to how your body reacts during conversations, notice how you breathe, and be aware of your body. You'll have more engaged and empathetic conversations this way. Manage and resolve conflicts with somatic strategies. Mindfulness breathing or grounding exercises can help keep you calm before a difficult conversation, allowing you to think more clearly and communicate more effectively.

Building a supportive environment

Make your living space somatically friendly. For example, you might create a space dedicated to meditation and exercise or arrange your work area to promote good posture and allow for movement breaks. Don't be afraid to share your practice with others. Organize group meditation sessions, do community yoga, or just share techniques with family and friends. Building a community around somatic practices can provide support and deepen your own commitment.

Making It Sustainable

Consider the impact of your somatic practices regularly. Have you noticed any benefits? How did you deal with challenges? Your practices can be reinforced and improved by reflection. It's important to adjust your somatic practices as your needs and circumstances change. Don't be afraid to try new things and toss out the ones that no longer work for you. This keeps your practice fresh and relevant to your life. Using somatic practices in your daily life transforms theoretical knowledge into practical, transformative actions. By shifting your lifestyle, you're not only improving your health, but you're also enhancing your relationships with others and your environment. Somatic practices, when practiced in this way, become more than just something you do, they become a part of who you are and how you live your life, and become a fundamental part of your identity.

Part 3

With somatic practices incorporated into everyday life, we now dig into how to create 'mindful moments'. These quick, on-the-go exercises develop somatic awareness while you're busy, offering practical methods to stay connected to your body and breath. With this approach, fleeting pauses become opportunities for mindfulness and rejuvenation.

THREE ON-THE-GO EXERCISES: MINDFUL MOMENTS

1. One-Minute Breathing Space

When to use it - To calm down after a stressful interaction, before an important meeting, or when overwhelmed with work. Making a difficult decision or transitioning between tasks to ensure you're thinking clearly.

How to do it - You can do it anywhere, just focus on your breathing for a minute. Breathe deeply through your nose, expanding your belly, then exhale slowly through your mouth. If possible, close your eyes and focus more on your breathing.

Benefits - This exercise helps reset your nervous system, reduces stress, and refocuses your mind, making it especially useful during transitions between different tasks or before starting a new activity.

2. Sensory Check-In

When to use it - Virtually anywhere. When you're on your break, at your desk, in a park, or even while commuting.

How to do it - Take a moment and engage all your senses. Note one thing you can see, one thing you can hear, and one thing you can touch. Just observe what's going on around you without judgment.

Benefits - The practice improves your sensory awareness and helps you maintain a more mindful relationship with your surroundings, which often helps you relax from mental stress.

3. Gratitude Stretch

When to use it - Again virtually anywhere. At home in a quiet setting or at work. Before or after a workout at a gym.

How to do it - Take a deep breath in and stretch your arms overhead. As you exhale and lower your arms, think of one thing you are grateful for at that moment. Try this stretch a few times, focusing on a different aspect of gratitude each time.

187

Benefits - Combining physical stretching with gratitude boosts your body's energy and stimulates your emotions, leading to a happier, healthier mindset.

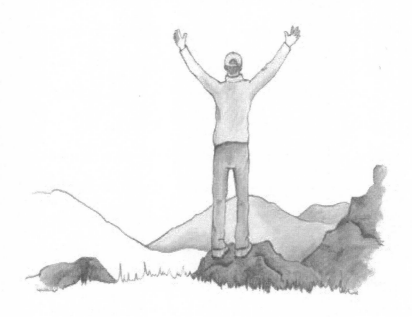

It's all about finding the extraordinary in the ordinary during mindful moments. There's nothing special about them, they're quick and accessible and you can do them anywhere, anytime. From waiting in line at the grocery store to sitting at your desk, these exercises can fit any time of day. Use routine breaks as opportunities to reconnect with your body and breath, turning them into mini mindfulness sessions. Use your phone or computer to set regular reminders or link them to habitual stuff like drinking water or checking emails. Slowly, these mindful pauses can become part of your daily routine, enhancing your overall somatic awareness and helping you become more present.

As you incorporate mindfulness into your daily schedule, you grow in somatic awareness and gain the capacity to engage fully and calmly with life's challenges and opportunities. The practice is fundamental to living a somatic lifestyle, turning brief, everyday actions into significant growth opportunities.

CHAPTER 11

Part 1

EXPLORING DIVERSE SOMATICS PRACTICES

To understand what somatics are all about, we need to look at the varied therapeutic methods in this field. One of the best techniques for processing trauma is Eye Movement Desensitization and Re-processing (EMDR). Body movement and mental health go hand-in-hand, illustrating the versatility and depth of somatic therapies.

EMDR Eye Movement Desensitization and Re-processing

People who have PTSD, anxiety, depression, or panic problems can benefit from EMDR; a psycho-therapy technique that helps them recover from traumas. A key feature of EMDR is bilateral stimu-lation - usually through guided eye movements - that physically activates the brain's processing path-ways.

190

In EMDR therapy, there are eight phases. The first is the history-taking session, during which the therapist assesses your readiness for treatment. The second is preparation. The therapist makes sure you know several ways to handle emotional distress and teaches you about EMDR. They explain what they'll do and establish trust. Phase three is about assessment. In this phase, the therapist finds the vivid visual image from the memory, the negative belief about yourself, and the emotions and sensations associated with it. The therapist will also help you choose a positive belief. Phase four is desensitization. During this phase, eye movements and bilateral stimulation are used while you focus on the trauma memory. The therapist will guide your eyes with their hand. Five is installation. You're trying to strengthen the positive belief that you'd want to replace the negative one. Phase six is body scan. Your therapist will ask you to hold the positive belief while you scan your body for residual tension or unusual sensations, which are then reprocessed. Phase seven is closure. Whether the reprocessing is complete or not, this phase gets you back to balance. And phase eight is re-evaluation. The therapist reviews progress and verifies that the results have been maintained and assesses if other target memories need to be reprocessed.

Your eye movements mimic Rapid Eye Movement (REM) sleep, which is associated with processing emotions and memories. The EMDR technique can help you deal with trauma faster than traditional talk therapy. In many cases, EMDR therapy reduces the vividness and emotional charge of trauma memories. You often find a greater sense of emotional stability and better mental health after processing distressing memories. Healing with EMDR emphasizes the role of the body in mental health. A lot of EMDR therapists include physical movement to increase bilateral stimulation, such as tapping or alternating hand clapping, which further engages the body. You can prepare yourself physically and mentally for EMDR by practicing deep breathing, mindfulness, or gentle yoga. Following an EMDR session, you may benefit from somatic awareness techniques to help integrate your experiences and ground yourself, especially if the memory processing evokes strong physical sensations or emotions.

The use of EMDR therapy illustrates how somatic practices can boost mental health strategies. Through EMDR, it becomes clear how the body's movements and the brain's health are deeply connected, each influencing the other in healing and growth. EMDR, because of this perspective, not only contributes to trauma recovery but also increases our understanding of how somatic therapies can affect our lives in positive ways.

Part 2

Based on the understanding of EMDR as a powerful method for trauma processing, we turn our attention to another significant approach within the realm of somatic practices known as Somatic Experiencing

(SE). Dr. Peter Levine developed this therapy based on the observation that wild animals are rarely traumatized despite regular threats. Instead, they use innate mechanisms to regulate and discharge the high levels of energy arousal associated with survival. It's these mechanisms that help the release of traumatic shock, which helps transform trauma.

SOMATIC EXPERIENCING

Somatic Experiencing provides a methodical approach to resolving the symptoms of trauma. According to SE, trauma symptoms are caused by a stressed nervous system that can't relax. It happens when someone's natural fight, flight, or freeze responses are thwarted during trauma. People learn to track their bodily sensations through SE and are guided to develop increased tolerance for difficult bodily sensations. SE teaches you to become aware of your bodily sensations to help them manage states of arousal associated with trauma.

It's different from traditional therapy, which primarily emphasizes recalling memories and activating emotions. SE focuses on bodily experiences to release tension. The benefits of SE are clear. PTSD, anxiety, depression, and more are all relieved. People feel empowered, by regaining control of their bodies and emotions. Stress-coping skills are often improved, and practitioners report increased resilience. How is it done? To start, the therapist creates a safe, supportive environment. You're then encouraged to slowly become aware of how you're feeling, and what you're feeling. It's not about recounting traumatic events in detail. Together, you and your therapist track your sensations and identify areas of discomfort or tension. Increasing your capacity to handle bodily sensations and emotions slowly is key. By identifying relaxation and mild distress sensations, you can help yourself pendulate between them. In SE, pendulation helps the nervous system regain its ability to self-regulate by moving between regulation and dysregulation.

195

Therapists use gentle prompts to help you explore your physical sensations and encourage movements that were repressed or unfulfilled during the traumatic event. During this process, the therapist makes sure you don't feel overwhelmed. Techniques such as grounding are used to help maintain stability. Grounding techniques help to keep you present in your body. You can incorporate SE into your daily life by regularly scanning your body to stay grounded and catch early signs of distress. Exercises like mindful walking, deep belly breathing, or physical grounding (feeling your feet on the ground) help maintain a calm and balanced nerve system.

With somatic experiencing therapy, trauma is treated by focusing on bodily sensations instead of its story. Among the fundamental elements of somatic practices, this method emphasizes the body's inherent wisdom and ability to heal itself. The more we explore SE along with other somatic techniques, the more we appreciate the power of our bodies to guide us through healing and make us feel alive. Having this understanding enhances the quality of our journey, and it enhances our understanding of health on a larger scale.

Part 3

It becomes clear as we examine the transformative effects of EMDR and Somatic Experiencing that these therapies offer not only insights, but also practical ways of healing and taking care of yourself. To further enhance their use, this section introduces three on-the-go exercises that incorporate EMDR and Somatic Experiencing into people's everyday lives. Designed to help maintain well-being, these exercises are quick, easy, and effective.

THREE ON-THE-GO EXERCISES FOR EMDR AND SOMATIC EXPERIENCING

1. Bilateral Tapping

When to use it - You can use this anywhere. Whether at home or work. It's discreet.

How to do it - Use your fingers to tap gently tap your thighs or arms while seated or standing. Think of something neutral or positive and keep a rhythm. A session should last about a minute or two.

Benefits - Reducing symptoms of anxiety and stress, this exercise uses bilateral stimulation, which is an aspect of EMDR.

2. Four Elements Breathing

When to use it - Exercises like this can be done anywhere, whether at home, at work, or outside, so they're easy to incorporate into your daily routine.

How to do it - You need to find a quiet and safe place and close your eyes. Let's imagine that each breath is a cycle of earth, water, air, and fire. As you inhale and exhale, visualize these elements moving through your body, each bringing a different healing quality or strength.

Benefits - Breathing this way helps unite the body and mind, enhancing internal harmony and helping with emotion processing. It's especially useful after stressful or triggering events.

3. Quick Coherence Technique

When to use it - In any setting, whether at work, home, or in public, you can use this technique for immediate stress relief.

How to do it - Focus on your breath with your hand over your heart. Imagine breathing in calm and breathing out tension. Become more relaxed by slowing down and deepening your breath.

Benefits - Reduced Stress, Improved Emotional Regulation, Enhanced Clarity and

Focus, Increased Resilience, Better Heart Health and a boosted Immune System.

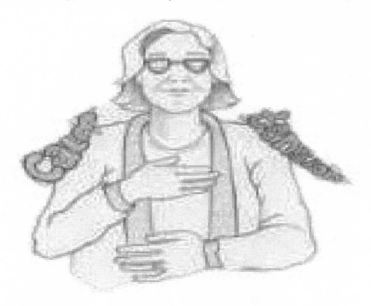

These exercises provide quick relief and build strength. They're especially helpful during stressful times or whenever you need a little Zen (relax and not worry about things that you cannot change). As you do these exercises regularly, you'll keep receiving the healing benefits of EMDR and Somatic Experiencing, enhancing your emotional and physical health. As we continue to explore somatic practices, these exercises serve as vital tools for maintaining balance, promoting healing, and enhancing one's capacity to handle life's challenges with strength and awareness.

CHAPTER 12

Part 1

EXPLORING DIVERSE SOMATIC PRACTICES
CONTINUED

Continuing our exploration of somatic practices, we explore the Feldenkrais Method, an
approach to understanding human movement and its
potential to promote change. Known for enhancing
self-awareness through movement and attention,
the Feldenkrais Method reduces pain and improves
physical function, as well as enhancing overall well-
being

The Feldenkrais Method

Developed by Moshe Feldenkrais, a physicist, judo
expert, and mechanical engineer, the Feldenkrais
Method is based on the synergy of insights from
physics, biomechanics, and psychology to provide
gentle movements and mindfulness to improve a
person's mental and physical health.

Rather than pushing for a specific result or posture correction, Feldenkrais focuses on how to move more freely and easily. By taking notice of your habitual neuromuscular patterns and rigidities, you can expand options for new ways of moving, while increasing sensitivity and efficiency.

Awareness Through Movement (ATM) - Teachers guide students verbally through a series of movement explorations that involve thinking, sensing, moving, and imagining. Small movements are practiced with little effort and without pain. In this class, the moves are usually performed lying on the floor, sitting, or standing, and they are exploratory in nature, allowing students to discover new movements and become more aware of themselves.

Functional Integration (FI) - These one-on-one lessons are tailored to meet the specific needs and preferences of each student, which involves gentle touching and manipulation by the teacher to guide the student into a range of motions which promote increased awareness of their bodies as well as improved motor control.

Each approach focuses on learning to feel comfortable with one's own body and movements, improving flexibility, coordination, and discovering one's natural capacity for graceful, efficient movement. We use non-invasive methods to change movement habits and posture that can cause or contribute to discomfort.

The benefits of the Feldenkrais Method

Improved Self-Awareness and Well-being - The experience often enhances mental and physical flexibility and redefines what it means to live in your body.

Pain Reduction - The trick to easing overused or strained muscles is to move more gently and efficiently.

Increased Range of Motion and Flexibility - As a result, students tend to find an increased range of motion and ease in their movements.

203

Using the Feldenkrais Method in your Daily Life

Feldenkrais principles can be incorporated into everyday activities, such as sitting, standing, and walking. Be aware of how you move during these activities to reduce strain and increase comfort. Take part in regular Awareness through Movement sessions, whether that's online classes, recordings, or group sessions, so you're always conscious of your body. Explore new hobbies or sports by applying Feldenkrais principles to learn more efficiently and effectively.

When we embrace the Feldenkrais Method, we gain not just a technique for improving ourselves, but a philosophy of movement that encourages a curious, kind approach to our bodies. Not only does this method challenge our movement habits, but it also improves our overall health and vitality. As a result of Feldenkrais, we learn the profound connection between what we do and what we think and feel, empowering us to live a more harmonious life.

204

Part 2

Following Feldenkrais, we move on to another deep somatic practice: Hakomi. Developed by Ron Kurtz in the 1970s, the Hakomi Method is a form of mindful somatic psychology that combines Western psychology and Eastern philosophies. In this approach, self-study, mindfulness, and the body's knowledge are the key to healing, growth, and transformation.

THE HAKOMI METHOD

The Hakomi method uses mindfulness as a central tool to explore how we organize our experiences and access our internal resources. The gentle, yet powerful approach is based on the idea that there are "core materials" within people - memories, images, beliefs, neuronal patterns, and deeply rooted emotional dispositions - that lie beneath the level of awareness but have a significant impact on your behavior and attitude.

Understanding the Hakomi Method

Principles of Nonviolence and Mindfulness - A central principle of Hakomi is nonviolence, accepting people as they are without forcing them to change. This creates a safe therapeutic space. During therapy, mindfulness enhances your ability to be open, curious, and aware of your thoughts and feelings, leading to deeper insight and self-understanding, allowing you to explore vulnerable parts of your identity without feeling threatened.

Use of Experiments - In Hakomi, therapeutic experiments are conducted in mindfulness. These are small acts or gestures that help you uncover unconscious beliefs or memories, like inviting you to notice your reaction when a certain touch or movement is introduced.

Harmonizing body and mind - Methods like this focus on somatic aspects to get in touch with your consciousness. Bodily expressions, tensions, and postures expose beliefs and habits concerning your identity.

206

Benefits of the Hakomi Method

Enhanced Self-Awareness and Self-Discovery-
With compassion and curiosity, you'll often get
profound insights into your mind and emotions.

Resolution of Internal Conflicts - You can solve
conflicts and remove obstacles by recognizing and
changing fundamental issues.

Better Control of Emotions - Mindfulness and body
awareness help you to regulate your emotions more
effectively, helping your mental health and relationships.

Applying Hakomi in everyday life

Daily Mindfulness Practice - By incorporating mindfulness into our daily routines, we can enhance the self-awareness that we gain through Hakomi therapy. Mindful eating, walking, or communicating can help you feel more present and connected to the moment.

Self-Study Exercises - Explore your reactions and behaviors through self-reflection and journaling. This can be seen as an extension of the 'experiments' used in Hakomi therapy, helping to reveal personal patterns and beliefs.

Body Awareness Routines - You can maintain Hakomi's effectiveness with simple routines like yoga, tai chi, and mindful stretching. These practices support the body's contribution to psychological health and personal development.

Getting into the details of the Hakomi Method reveals another layer of somatic practices. By using this method, we not only learn how the mind and body interact, but we also get practical tools for

making significant life changes. By using mindfulness and body awareness, the Hakomi Method encourages psychological healing as well às self-discovery and connection.

Part 3

Based on the exploration of Feldenkrais and
Hakomi methods, it's clear these somatic practices
not only deepen our understanding of body awareness, but also provide practical, accessible tools for
everyday life. These on-the-go exercises blend
Hakomi and Feldenkrais principles to help you apply these skills in daily life. These exercises are designed to be quick and effective so won't take too
much time, helping to promote mindfulness, flexibility, and self-awareness throughout your day.

THREE ON-THE-GO EXERCISES
INCORPORATING THE FELDENKRAIS AND
HAKOMI METHOD

1. Mindful Pause

When to use it - At your desk, in your car, before or after commuting, at home in a quiet space, in a public park, before entering stressful environments like meeting rooms, and at a library.

How to do it - Stop whatever you're doing, take three deep breaths, and feel the sensations in your body. Put a lot of focus on any tension or discomfort. With each exhale, picture telling your breath to go to these areas, inviting them to relax.

Benefits - It helps with emotional regulation and stress management because it's based on Hakomi's mindfulness aspect.

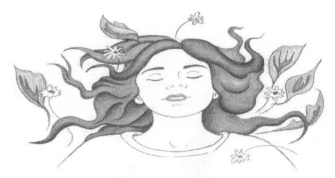

2. Feldenkrais Pelvic Tilt Mini-Session

When to use it - Lie down or sit comfortably any-where that's calm and private, like at home on a mat or in a chair, during a time out at work, at a fitness or wellness center, or while traveling in a hotel room.

How to do it - Rock your pelvis forward and back-ward slowly while you're sitting in your office chair or even on public transport if you feel comfortable. You'll notice subtle changes in your spine and lower back. Don't overdo it, just stay focused on the sen-sation you get from each small and controlled movement. Inhale and gently push your pelvis back-ward, which will naturally arch your lower back slightly and push your stomach forward. Exhale and roll your pelvis forward, flattening your lower back

211

against the back of the chair, as if trying to tuck your tailbone under. Ensure each movement is smooth and controlled.

Benefits - Over time, this Feldenkrais-inspired exercise gradually helps to improve and realign your posture. This is especially helpful for people who spend many hours seated, as it helps alleviate the stiffness and discomfort that often result from extended periods in a chair.

3. Peripheral Awareness Expansion

When to use it - At an office desk to reduce mental fatigue, outside in a park to enhance environmental connection, at home in a quiet room for relaxation, or in public spaces like cafes or waiting areas where you can focus safely.

How to do it - Stand or sit and focus on a point directly in front of you. Gradually widen your field of vision so you can see as far as you can, what's on both sides of your head without moving your eyes. Observe what you can see and feel and hold that awareness for a moment. The goal is not to strain your eyes but to relax and allow the information to come to you. Coordinate your breathing with your expanding awareness. Inhale deeply as you focus on expanding your sight and exhale as you relax deeper into the awareness of your surroundings and body.

Benefits - This exercise, which uses Hakomi's principles of expanding consciousness, can help you become more aware of your surroundings and calm your nerves.

These exercises are designed to fit smoothly into your daily routine, offering methods to improve mindfulness and body awareness without interrupting your schedule. It only takes a few minutes to engage in these practices, whether you're commuting, at work, or at home. Just a couple minutes of these exercises throughout the day can have a big impact. You can make these exercises a regular part of your day by tying them to daily habits like drinking coffee or taking a break.

As we explore and apply the principles of the Feldenkrais and Hakomi methods into our lives, these exercises offer immediate relief and comfort, while also deepening our somatic awareness and enhancing overall health. It is this approach that enables us to make each day a more immersive experience as we move through life with greater ease and presence.

CHAPTER 13

Part 1

FURTHER EXPANSION OF YOUR SOMATIC TOOLKIT

We've come to the end of our journey exploring somatic practices, and we've learnt how awareness and movement make a big difference to our health. Further adding the Alexander Technique to our toolkit gives us new ways to improve how we use ourselves in everyday activities. By learning balance, posture, and movement in everyday life, this method helps us unlearn bad habits that cause physical and mental stress.

The Alexander Technique

Around the 1890s, Frederick Matthias Alexander developed the Alexander Technique, which teaches people to stop using unnecessary muscles and mental tension during their everyday lives. This simple approach improves ease of movement, balance, support, and coordination.

215

Using this technique, you'll use the right amount of energy for each activity. This isn't a series of treatments or exercises but rather a re-education of the mind and body toward greater self-awareness.

At its core, the Alexander Technique changes long-standing habits that cause unnecessary tension. It emphasizes the head, neck, and spine relationship, which determines how we function. Using gentle hands-on guidance and verbal instructions, the method helps students find ease and balance in simple movements and daily activities like sitting, standing, walking, and bending. The benefits of this therapy include better posture, reduced back pain, and alleviation of chronic stiffness. Performing artists like musicians and actors find it improves stamina, accuracy, and clarity of perception.

Changing long-standing habits takes practice and patience, so practice and patience are essential. Here are easy ways to put its principles into practice:

Mindfulness in Motion - Check your posture and alignment regularly. Do you slump when you sit? When you look at your computer screen, do you tense your neck? Even small adjustments can make a big difference.

Conscious Control - Whenever you do anything, think about how you can do it more comfortably. If you're standing up, think about the sequence of movements and consciously engage your muscles smoothly.

Constructive Rest - Get some rest during the day. Lay on the floor with your knees bent and your head supported, releasing tension and stretching your spine.

The Alexander Technique not only adds to our somatic toolkit but also gives us a philosophy of movement that fits seamlessly into our daily lives. It's just a matter of monitoring what you do and how you do it. Through this technique, we're constantly learning and unlearning, making sure our movements and postures contribute to our overall health

217

instead of detracting from it. With the Alexander Technique, we can create a life of ease and well-being, where every movement is an opportunity to improve balance and self-awareness.

Part 2

After learning the Alexander Technique's attention to movement and posture, we'll switch to another transformational somatic practice: Body-Mind Centering. Bonnie Bainbridge Cohen developed BMC, which explores the connection between mind and body through movement, touch, voice, and thought. This practice combines scientific understanding with insights from psychological and spiritual disciplines, improving physical and emotional well-being.

BODY-MIND CENTERING

This approach uses hands-on methods, movement, and voice work to teach you about your body, such as your skeleton and muscles, to improve co-ordination. It also investigates how we develop from before birth through early childhood, showing how this knowledge can transform your movements and overall health. You'll learn to spot and change limiting behaviors and movements, which increases your flexibility and awareness. Understanding your body better can also improve how you communicate and connect with others, and studying how you developed can help you understand your emotions and behaviors from early on.

Applying Body-Mind Centering in Everyday Life

Your daily routine should include BMC exercises that target specific systems. Start your day with fluid spine movements to boost spinal health or diaphragmatic breathing (deep breathing) to relax your core. Try crawling and rolling, which are simple developmental movements. It's a fun way to refresh the neuromuscular system and reconnect with foundational movement patterns. Explore different body tissues through touch, such as muscles, bones, organs, and fluids. Whether you do it alone or with a partner, it helps you gain a deeper understanding of your body.

In our exploration of Body-Mind centering as part of our Somatic toolkit, we learn how physically and mentally connected we are. BMC helps us heal and change and deepens our understanding and connection with our bodies and minds as active, interrelated parts of who we are. Through BMC, we learn to not just exist in our bodies but to actively engage

220

with them, experiencing the world with fresh energy and vitality.

Part 3

Building on our exploration of the Alexander Technique and Body-Mind Centering, we now introduce three practical on-the-go exercises that reflect the core principles of these methods. The exercises are simple and easy to do, so you can easily incorporate somatic awareness into your day-to-day.

THREE ON-THE-GO EXERCISES INCORPORATING THE ALEXANDER TECHNIQUE AND BODY-MIND CENTERING

1. Constructive Rest for the Alexander Technique

When to use it - This is perfect for any quiet, comfortable space where you can lie down. At home, in a yoga or fitness studio, in a private office, or a park or garden.

How to do it - Find a quiet spot where you can lie on your back with your knees bent and feet flat on the floor. If you need it, put a book or cushion under your head. Let your hands rest on your belly.

222

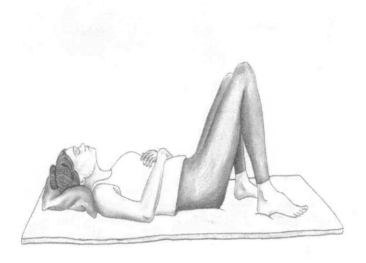

Shut your eyes and spend 10-15 minutes concentrating on relaxing your body, beginning at your neck and progressing down to your feet.

Benefits - Helps reduce muscle tension, align the spine, and promote a relaxed state in both body and mind, reflecting the Alexander Technique's emphasis on improving overall physiological function through relaxation and proper alignment.

223

2. Embodied Anatomy Exploration for Body-Mind Centering

When to use it - A quiet room at home, a dance studio, a secluded park, or a workshop or retreat center.

How to do it - Make a daily choice (like bone, muscle, or organ). Bring it to your attention as you go about your day. For example, focus on your bones and notice how your skeleton feels during various activities. Notice how being aware changes your movement and posture.

Benefits - The practice helps you appreciate how each part of your body supports the others, leading to more mindful and efficient movement.

3. Mindful Movement Integration

When to use it - At home, outside in a park, in a gym or fitness studio, or at the office if you have a private or quiet area during breaks.

How to do it - Throughout the day, as you walk, sit, or stand, slow down and pay attention to how your body moves. Identify any unnecessary tensions, especially in your neck and shoulders, and let them go. Neck rolls, shoulder shrugs, and stretches can relieve tension.

Benefits - This exercise blends principles from both the Alexander Technique and Body Mind Centering by developing an awareness of movement patterns that promote physical ease and efficiency. This helps you unlearn harmful posture habits and adopt a more relaxed, aligned posture.

These exercises are designed to easily fit into your daily routine, requiring no special equipment or setting, making them ideal for busy on-the-go lifestyles. By practicing these exercises regularly, you can slowly build a deeper awareness of your body that improves both your physical and mental health. At least one of these exercises should be a part of your daily routine, perhaps Constructive Rest in the morning or Mindful Movement Integration as you move around.

Spend a few minutes after each exercise reflecting on any changes you noticed in yourself. Reflecting on the exercises can make them resonate more deeply and help you connect with their principles. These practical exercises connect the ideas of the Alexander Technique and Body-Mind Centering with their everyday uses. As well as improving physical harmony and reducing tension, they also affect mental and emotional balance, promoting a holistic sense of well-being.

CONCLUSION

As we draw this exploration to a close, it's valuable to reflect on the journey we've shared through somatic therapy and its capacity for transformation. From foundational theories to whole practices, this book shows how somatic methods improve health.

When it comes to trauma, stress, and tension, the mind and body are linked. From self-awareness exercises to EMDR and Somatic Experiencing, the introduction to various somatic practices shows there are a lot of ways to nurture a healthy body and mind. We can take away that awareness - both self-awareness and sensory awareness - is key to healing. By becoming more aware of our body's subtle cues, we can manage stress and even prevent it. We talked about various methods, like Qigong and EFT Tapping, to highlight the advantages of a holistic approach to health. The emphasis on 'on-the-go' exercises shows how somatic therapy is practical, adaptable, and can be easily added to daily routines, offering sustainable health benefits beyond crisis management. In exploring communal practices, we find that social support often leads to deeper and more sustained healing. Finally, healing is framed as a lifelong journey, with somatic practices serving as an ongoing resource for personal growth and development.

As you move forward, let this book be a reminder that learning about somatic awareness is a continuous process, constantly deepening your connection to yourself and your surroundings. Keep an open mind as you explore both familiar and new techniques, embracing the experiences and insights that come your way.

"The body is the doorway, not the obstacle. Through our physical selves, we access experiences richer than words, theories, and fears can describe. Within this depth, we uncover the significant healing and transformative power of somatic practices."

It is my hope that this journey inspires you to explore, engage, and embrace the wisdom of your body, so you can heal and understand yourself better. Wishing your health, healing, and happiness as your body and mind continue to work together.

Thanks for reading

I enjoyed writing this book, and I truly hope you've enjoyed it too. It has been scary at times, but I believe I've done a great job. If possible, could you leave a review on Amazon? I'd appreciate it! Your feedback is so important to me and lets me know how I've done and what I can improve on in my next book which is going to be on self-help again.

Simply scan this QR code with your phone, and you will be taken to the book's review page.

Alternatively, to leave a review:

Head over to the book's page on Amazon or find it through your purchases

Scroll down towards the bottom of the page and click on the button that says "Write a Customer Review"

You can simply leave a star rating out of 5 or write a short review!

AUTHORS AFTERTHOUGHT

As I wrote the words "As we draw this exploration to a close", I shed a tear.

This book has been a friend to me and it's quite sad now it's over.

My reason for writing this book was to raise money to help a friend with multiple sclerosis get the treatment he desperately needs.

This is still a goal for me, but I think success looks like someone not having to deal with what he deals with every day.

I truly hope at least one person takes value from it as much as he does. Yes, some exercises (pretty much all) are easy, but they have such a huge impact.

I truly believe Somatics is the answer!

Jess x

Made in United States
Orlando, FL
30 October 2024